# OPERATING IN THE DARK

# OPERATING IN THE DARK

## The Accountability Crisis in Canada's Health Care System

*Lisa Priest*

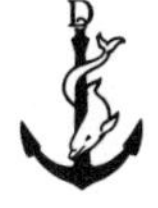

Doubleday Canada Limited

**Canadian Cataloguing in Publication Data**

Priest, Lisa, 1964–
Operating in the Dark

Includes index.

ISBN 0-385-25719-8

1. Medicare care—Canada. I. Title.

RA399.C3P74 1998 362.1'0971 C98-931223-2

Jacket design by Joseph Gisani, Andrew Smith Graphics
Jacket photo courtesy Dick Loek/*Toronto Star*
Text design by Heidy Lawrance Associates
Printed and bound in the USA

Published in Canada by
Doubleday Canada Limited
105 Bond Street
Toronto, Ontario
M5B 1Y3

BVG 10 9 8 7 6 5 4 3 2 1

*In memory of my father,*
*Arthur Bernard Priest*

# Contents

# Acknowledgments

This project began with a simple question: Why can't I find out how good my hospitals and doctors are?

Although the question was a straightforward one, the answers were not. This book project was exhaustive and could not have come to fruition if the topic had not first been selected as a worthy public policy issue to be probed for the 1996-97 Atkinson Fellowship in Public Policy. The Atkinson Charitable Foundation's generous support gave me a full year to travel, research, and write about the lack of accountability in Canada's health care system. Special thanks go to John Honderich, Charles Pascal, and Beland Honderich for believing in the project, in addition to other members of the selection committee. In those early stages, research assistant Dawn Calleja, Freedom of Information researcher Ken Rubin, Adele Jushka at the Foundation, and editors Joe Hall, Alan Marshall, and Peter Gorrie of the *Toronto Star*, all contributed to the successful completion of the project, which appeared as a lengthy newspaper series in the *Toronto Star*.

That would have been the end of this project had agent Helen Heller and Doubleday Editor-in-Chief John Pearce not agreed with me that the material required further research and expansion into a book. They also gave considerable editorial advice, offering suggestions on the manuscript, as did others at Doubleday. Pamela Murray, in particular, was a great help in the later stages of the editorial process. Editor Jennifer Glossop was immensely helpful with structure; if there was a guide to best book editors, she would most certainly be in it.

More than 150 people gave generously of their time as interview subjects, providing research studies and direction on policies. While some of them may not agree with this book's conclusions, I am nevertheless grateful for their participation. Although I cannot mention them all by name, there are a few who stand out: Duncan Sinclair for his policy advice; my fiancé, Dr. Geoff Anderson, for his insight and advice, and for sharing his study on hospital downsizing; Dr. Paul Walker for helping design a hospital survey; and Dr. Alan Hudson and Michael Decter for providing good advice and a helping hand whenever needed. Peter Ellis not only provided me with insight into England's health care system, he generously helped arrange interviews overseas. Ron Marston allowed me to follow him through the waiting list and operation for a double-knee replacement, and many other patients gave of their time and spoke of their experiences. Barb Priest's wizardry with spreadsheets helped me understand survey results. Crown attorney Christina Kopynsky generously provided me with inquest materials. Lawyer Ray Flett was also of great help.

Finally, I would like to thank Geoff, for his love, patience and understanding during a seemingly endless project that took up most of my days and nights.

# Preface

For years, I kept getting the same phone-calls. People telephoned me at the *Toronto Star*, where I work as a health reporter, relating stories of suspected medical malpractice. They were desperate, some of them in pain, almost all of them frightened of what the future held.

Initially, I was keen to do stories on these victims of medical malpractice and those who had relatives who had mysteriously died while in hospital, but after a while there were so many letters, so many complaints, it would have taken dozens of reporters to sift through these medical mishaps. When I did try to tackle one of these stories, hospital officials were not keen to comment, and without documentation it often became the word of a patient against that of the powerful medical establishment, leaving little doubt as to who was going to win. Overwhelmed by the number of calls and letters I had received, I filed most of them in my cabinet in a brown paper envelope with the word "victims" scrawled on it, promising myself I would get back to these people some day in the future.

At the same time, people called to say they had just been diagnosed or knew of someone who needed an operation or other medical treatment, but they didn't know how to locate the best specialist or hospital. They were facing the most important decisions of their lives and they had no information on where to go, what to do, or whom to call. I became their last hope in a series of desperate queries. They were women with breast cancer, elderly men with heart disease, mothers worried about their children, those languishing on waiting lists, patients who had been injured during surgery only to be bounced from one specialist to another. They believed there must be someone somewhere who could point them in the right direction. These were informed, bright, savvy health care consumers who were justifiably reluctant to turn over their most prized possessions—their bodies—with no questions asked. They wanted more hard facts and fewer godlike figures who claimed to have the solutions but not necessarily all of the answers. Who is the best heart surgeon? How do I find the shortest wait for my hip replacement? How can I ensure I get my radiation treatment in a timely fashion? They were all good questions, and I didn't have all the answers.

Although I knew some of the "bests" in health care, it was by reputation only—hardly a substitute for the consumer guides to hospitals and doctors in the United States. Some of the callers were appalled by my lack of information, but many more were surprised, wondering how I could deal with medical experts all day long but not have a mental, ready-to-go Rolodex of the "bests." That made me wonder why we, as taxpayers, fund a medical system for more than $76 billion a year, yet have so little information on how well its institutions and individuals perform. How is it that patients can pay every penny into a system, but not have an ounce of power in it? Why is there no consumer guide that tells patients where to get the best, most competent care as there is with hotels and restaurants? And wouldn't disclosure of that kind of information make the system safer by forcing the weak spots to get fixed?

Yet from my conversations with doctors, I knew they were feeling beaten down and unappreciated, victims of a tight-fisted government that was trying to control health spending and was keen on costs, not on quality of care. For most of them, being measured on performance was just another attempt by government to attack them, rate them, control how and where they could practise medicine. To aggravate matters, they had heard stories of doctors in the United States who had been unfavourably reviewed in the popular press, only to lose their positions or be kindly told to move on. The prospect of being measured was frightening and many doctors were in favour of the status quo, at least until the perfect method was found to rate them.

In spring 1996, an application for the Atkinson Fellowship in Public Policy was posted on the *Star* bulletin board. I applied for it, suggesting in about five thousand words how the lack of accountability in the health care system needed to be researched. My proposal began with this simple, yet important, question: Why can we learn more when looking for a garage mechanic than when shopping for a hospital? If I had not won that fellowship and its year of research funding from the Atkinson Charitable Foundation, I might never have had the opportunity to explore the issues behind that simple query. Thanks to the fellowship funding, I travelled to England, to the United States, and coast to coast in Canada, and was able to dig deep into a difficult, unexplored area.

The resulting newspaper series "Operating in the Dark" appeared in the *Toronto Star* in the fall of 1997, and the reaction ranged from very positive to extraordinarily negative. There was a predictable firestorm of protest from members of the Ontario Medical Association, which included e-mail from doctors who called me a "malignant ignoramus" and a "bitch," and one who said he would not treat me if I had a bad-prognosis melanoma.

Many others in health care felt that the series was long overdue, and they were eager to take part in helping to make the health care system more accountable—something they themselves had been trying to do in their own quiet way through research grants and hospital quality programs. Patients felt I had revealed the tip of an iceberg and they promptly pointed me to more areas they thought should be investigated. They were grateful their concerns had been legitimized and felt empowered to start asking some tough questions of the medical establishment and hospitals.

Exciting things began to happen. The Ontario

Hospital Association moved to create hospital report cards; academics are being funded to create a national scorecard; and the Atkinson Charitable Foundation awarded a further grant to explore what it would take to create consumer guides on hospitals, doctors and community health services in Ontario, with an eye to expanding it across Canada. Other hospitals and groups are also doing their own individual report cards.

Despite the newspaper series' length, I felt there was more to be explored, new stories to tell, and areas where the lack of accountability on health care needed to be revealed and probed in the length of a book. Doubleday Editor-in-Chief John Pearce, whom I had met with a number of times in the past, had told me the only book he wanted me to write was on a subject I felt passionate about. This was the one.

This book is my attempt to empower and aid prospective health care consumers. That stack of mail in the brown envelope in my file drawer marked "victims" needed to be opened. For decades, health care consumers have been inadvertently shut out from the health care system because they have been intimidated by the elitist language, the white coats, and the complexity of their diseases or ailments.

This is also the book some members of the medical establishment don't want you to read, because it will make you question them, research them, and ultimately grab the power back from an old boys' club that, as patients, we were never invited to join.

# Introduction

Would you climb into a jet if you knew the pilots were not routinely tested for their ability to fly? Sounds like a crazy question. After all, no airline could exist if it didn't allow Transport Canada to regularly monitor its pilots and ensure the safety of its passengers. It's unthinkable. But that's much the way doctors and surgeons in Canadian hospitals work.

Unlike pilots, licensed doctors go through their entire careers without as much as a competency check, even though the life and death stakes are just as high. To take just one example, as an Airbus-320 captain, David Noble of Toronto had to go through about sixty competency checks in his career before his retirement. But except for the occasional testing here and there, particularly for physicians over seventy, the vast majority of doctors are not routinely checked on their abilities in the operating room or in their medical practices. Most of us would not hand over our car to a mechanic without making inquiries, or get our hair cut without a recommendation. Yet we hand more than $76 billion to a system with few checks and balances.

It shouldn't be that way. As a matter of informed consent, prospective patients should be able to learn not only the death and complication rates of an operation but those rates *in a particular surgeon's hands*. Being told the death rate for open heart surgery is three per cent in Canadian hospitals isn't comforting if the pair of hands opening your chest has a higher mortality track record in the operating room.

In many parts of the United States, patients are able to peruse state-created consumer guides that list risk-adjusted death rates by doctors' names. "Risk-adjusted death rates" means the numbers are adjusted for the severity of the risk associated with the patients, be they elderly, very ill, or complicated by other medical factors that would make their surgery and recovery less successful. This ensures that the ratings are fair and surgeons aren't unfairly judged if they operate on the sickest patients. As a result of these state-wide guides, the cardiac surgery death rates in New York state have dropped by fifty-two per cent over a five-year period, studies have shown.

This isn't to say that hospitals are dangerous places or that those who work in them are negligent. But if hospitals and doctors vary so much in the United States, and the publishing of that information has helped make things better, then the same positive changes could happen in Canada.

To understand how Canadians got to this point, some history is in order.

Even though our health care system, also called medicare, is over three decades old, many Canadians forget it was a social program that took several decades to build. The first promise to build a form of national health insurance came from Mackenzie King in 1919, but it was a Saskatchewan man with an unsettling medical experience in his youth who really pioneered what we now know as medicare. As a boy in Winnipeg, Tommy Douglas developed a bone infection in his leg and his doctor recommended amputation. Fortunately, Douglas got better and didn't have to lose his leg, but he was left with the impression that his care wasn't as good as it should have been because he had been a public, not a private, patient. When he entered politics, Douglas began to champion an equal, equitable health care system for all Canadians, no matter how rich or poor. Two years after his Cooperative Commonwealth Federation came to power in 1944, Saskatchewan passed the Hospitalization Act, which provided public insurance for hospital care. Two years later, in 1948, the federal government got into the act by implementing the National Health Grant Program, almost all of which went to construct new hospitals. But it wasn't until almost a decade later, in 1957, that Parliament passed the Hospital Insurance and Diagnostic Services Act, which provided federal monies to any province that created its own hospital insurance program, provided those provinces meet a few criteria. The provinces had to administer the programs and provide comprehensive, universal care that was reasonably accessible to all residents and was portable enough that citizens from one province could be covered for medical services they had received in other provinces. That way, the provinces would fund essentially all the same medical services. Eventually all provinces joined the program and the federal government picked up the tab for half of the cost of services to hospitals.

As impressive as that move was, there was a basic problem: Costs for treating patients in doctor's offices were not covered under the legislation, prompting those who weren't sick enough to go to hospitals because they couldn't afford medical care any other way. Again, it was Tommy Douglas who led the way by devising the Saskatchewan Medical Care Insurance Act, legislation that angered physicians and prompted ninety per cent of them to go on strike in 1962. Despite the doctor's widespread disapproval, Douglas prevailed and Saskatchewan was not only the first province in Canada but the first jurisdiction in North America to have a tax-supported universal insurance program.

Things worked well over the next decade or so, but provinces and their health policy analysts were now wondering why so much money was going towards building new hospitals but not towards other programs such as home care, which was potentially much more efficient and less expensive. Health care providers wanted to experiment with new ways of delivering care, such as community and outpatient services, and in the mid-1970s Parliament passed the Established Programs Financing Act, which killed the

50-50 split in funding between the federal government and provinces. In its place, the federal government provided block funding for health and post-education programs. With that type of funding, provinces didn't have to explain exactly how they spent the money, provided it went to health and post-education.

But the health care system hit yet another obstacle in the early 1980s as concerns surfaced that patients without the cash couldn't get the same access to doctors who were "extra-billing" their patients. Although governments and provincial medical associations had negotiated fees for medical services, they weren't engraved in stone and doctors were able to charge extra. That certainly wasn't the accessible, universal health care system Douglas had had in mind, nor was it the one most Canadians had grown to love and revere as a crucial social program. In 1984, physician extra-billing was abolished by the Canada Health Act, which penalized any province that allowed physicians to charge above the negotiated fee agreed by government and medical associations. Although many doctors were angry at what they saw as an infringement on their rights, other doctors were dead set against extra-billing, saying it prevented those patients without money from getting the care they needed.

Extra-billing or user fees are still sometimes touted as a way to deter people from seeking unnecessary medical care. However, an often-quoted study refutes this argument. Two Canadian economists, Glen Beck and John Horne, tracked how forty thousand Saskatchewan families used health care from 1968, before these user fees were introduced, until 1971, when they were eradicated by that province's NDP government. They found that although provincial health costs were steady and there was a tiny drop in the use of physician services, the most vulnerable in society—the poor, the elderly, and those with large families—substantially decreased their use of health care services. Use of services by the poor fell by eighteen per cent alone. Conversely, middle-class patients saw doctors more frequently, particularly for services such as annual physical examinations.

Despite the extra-billing fight, the 1980s were still a time of great wealth as many hospitals saw eight per cent to double-digit increases in their budgets from provincial governments. When hospitals didn't balance their books, the government would bail them out, giving little incentive to balance budgets in the future. But the greedy 1980s gave way to the lean 1990s and governments, eager to control costs, used a two-pronged approach to achieve their aims: Reduce hospital costs and cap spending on physician services. The number of staffed beds dropped and hospitals began looking for more efficient ways to provide care. They found it by keeping patients in hospital for shorter periods of time. The average length of stay in short-term or acute-care hospitals dropped from nine days in 1986-87 to seven days in 1994-95, according to Statistics Canada figures. Although the length of stay dropped, many hospitals were treating more patients than ever.

Although cuts to hospitals have been substantial, overall funding of the health care system has remained relatively stable with Canadian health spending in 1997 forecast at $76.6 billion, which amounted to $2525 for every person in the country. Of that money, more than two-thirds is spent on the public system for hospitals, doctors, laboratory tests, and the like, with the other third going to the private sector for things such as prescription drugs, dental services, and semi-private coverage in hospital rooms.

Essentially, health care is paid for by federal and provincial tax dollars, but in recent years the federal government has cut its transfers to the provinces as part of its war on the deficit. Each province sets the amount it will spend on health. Hospitals have operating budgets, which provincial health ministries approve before cutting the cheques, but it's hospital administrators and in some provinces, regional health boards, who manage the costs and expenses of their institutions.

Canada's fifty-five thousand doctors are essentially independent. Most bill provincial health plans on a fee-for-service basis, which means physicians are paid for every medical procedure or treatment they provide. Many health care analysts have complained that this is an ineffective way to remunerate physicians, since it rewards doctors who do more procedures and pays some specialists who are trained for years to perform high-risk surgeries far less than those who have little risk and don't train for nearly as long. Generally speaking, brain surgeons are paid less than dermatologists; some doctors who treat those with the AIDS virus are paid less than general practitioners; and specialists who look after premature babies are not paid much more than family doctors. Geriatricians are paid the least of any specialty, and many say that unless they are put on salary at a hospital, they must do many other things besides treat elderly people to make a living. Although doctors as a group agree that some of their colleagues are not being paid as much as they should, paying them more inevitably means paying others less.

"The problem in Canada is that the process is left to the medical associations. It's very difficult to say, 'I'm overpaid,'" said Morris Barer, director of the Centre for Health Services and Policy Research at the University of British Columbia. Murray Mackenzie, chief executive officer of North York General Hospital in Toronto, has even stronger words, saying, "The whole fee schedule is insane. It needs to be tossed. There need to be massive adjustments on the fees. What should we look at? Social utility? Neonatologists and perinatologists [doctors who look after premature babies] are two of the lowest paid, but the benefits to the health care system are a great success story. What needs to be re-examined? Ophthalmologists, and cardiologists who get paid a lot for stress tests," said Mackenzie, answering his own question.

Another concern is what individual physicians make—something that is kept secret in every province except British Columbia, which has been publishing the annual billings of physicians to its health insurance plan for more than a quarter century, with little complaint. In Ontario, one has to apply through the Freedom of Information and Protection of Privacy Act (FOI) legislation to find out how much individual unidentified doctors bill the provincial health plan, as government still won't release this information.

An application through FOI legislation revealed that doctors in the same specialty bill the health insurance plan wildly differing amounts, with some billing three and four times what they are expected to for their specialty. In Metropolitan Toronto, for example, the top ten family doctors collectively billed the Ontario Health Insurance Plan $5.6 million in fiscal 1995-96. The top-billing general practitioner in Metro billed $663,010.79, more than four times the average billing of a family physician in Ontario in that same year. Obtaining that information took eight months and one appeal. The government didn't want to give out the figures, claiming they would be misleading. Some physicians who did not want their incomes disclosed even argued that "there was concern expressed regarding the personal safety of the doctors and their families if the information was disclosed."

Still, in Saskatchewan, where they are more open than Ontario but not nearly as forthcoming as British Columbia, one can quickly learn there are huge discrepancies. The annual statistical report of Saskatchewan Health found that one psychiatrist billed more than two-and-a-half times the average billing of those in his specialty, as did an obstetrician and otolaryngologist (ear and throat specialist). Trying to find out who these people are is impossible, as Saskatchewan Health refuses to say, nor can the names be obtained under the FOI legislation in that province.

British Columbia is the model of openness. It publishes the billings of doctors by name in a book each year simply because "we think the public has a right to know," said Martin Serediak, chair of the Medical Services Commission and assistant deputy minister of the Medical Services Plan in British Columbia. The west-coast province is also the only one in Canada to put a cap on the number of patients a family doctor can see in one day. A family doctor receives fifty per cent of fees for treating the forty-fifth to the sixty-second patient in one day, and after that receives no payment. Even if every patient was seen for as little as ten minutes, the doctor seeing sixty-two patients would have to work for more than ten hours a day. However, doctors do get fifteen per cent more per patient aged seventy-five and older, since these patients typically take longer to treat.

The amounts paid for certain procedures, particularly those that have not been proven to be effective, are also open to criticism. For example, in 1987-88 more than $900,000 worth of sleep studies were billed to the Ontario Health Insurance Plan (OHIP). Eight years later OHIP shelled out more than $17.6 million for similar studies in that one year—a twentyfold increase—even though "nobody knows the quality of the work," according to Dr. Gerald Gold, associate registrar of the College of Physicians and Surgeons of Ontario and director of quality management. One of the problems in medicine, Gold added, is that "a lot of so-called standards don't exist. In medicine, the majority of things done have not been validated through appropriate research."

Doctors have their own complaints about the system. Some don't feel they are paid enough or appreciated enough. Others complain that they have to ration health care services because funding is short in some areas, such as heart surgery and hip and knee replacement. Some involved in medical associations believe this is evidence that medicare is going broke and a private, parallel health care system is the way to help ease the burden on the tax-supported system. The thinking is that the extra cash on the private side would help ease up on the public system, which would provide "core medical services" to patients. Many health economists have disagreed with that assertion, saying there is more than enough cash in the system and the problem is how that money is being spent.

Medicare is not just any social program: It is the one Canadians revere, the one that defines and unites most of us in this vast country, making us the envy of many in the world. Although the government collects taxes and funds the health care system, it does not guarantee or monitor the quality of that care. In other words, the government may pay the bills, but it doesn't police the system. That job is left to the professions. Doctors claim to be self-policing but for the most part the colleges of physicians and surgeons in each province have largely been investigators of complaints, although some have been trying to break out of that mould by monitoring more physicians and setting up quality programs. The Canadian Council on Health Services Accreditation—the national body that accredits hospitals that volunteer to have it done for a fee—is assumed to act as the "Good Housekeeping seal of approval" for hospitals, but provides no help to patients trying to discern the quality of individual hospitals. However, it too is expected to implement report cards for hospitals in the future.

A crisis was inevitable. In the winter of 1998, the shortage of services in hospital emergency wards splashed horror stories on the front pages of newspapers and on the television news. Elderly patients were stacked on stretchers in the hospital halls. In Quebec City, the death of a sixty-five-year-old woman was blamed on Parti Québécois hospital budget cuts, as was the turning away of a rape victim in an emergency ward because of a staff shortage, though the latter case was later disputed. These troubling stories revealed there was a very real problem and to some it was further evidence that cuts were so deep in hospitals, they had gone past the bone and into the marrow.

There have been other crises in health care over the years. Ontario women with breast cancer who had surgery couldn't get timely radiation treatments afterwards, unless they wanted to travel hundreds of miles north and be away from their families for almost two months. Some women didn't want to be away for that long, so passed on the radiation treatment, which is given to help prevent a recurrence of cancer. A similar problem occurred with British Columbia men with prostate cancer who had to travel to the United States for their radiation treatment.

These shortages of services always get top billing by the media, and justifiably so, but some of those reading the newspapers and watching television assume, usually incorrectly, that this serves as further proof that there should be a private, parallel health care system. Linking a temporary shortage of services to the need for private care is a very large leap, as it assumes that the crisis of the day has to do with a lack of money, instead of a lack of adequate management of hospital resources. It's the medical equivalent of assuming that every headache is the symptom of a brain tumour.

Generally speaking, doctors who advocate two-tier care are frequently middle-aged or older and have noticed less care available for their patients over a period of decades. These are the doctors who have seen the most dramatic changes to the system in terms of cut beds, reduced operating room time, and longer waiting lists, which suggests to them that there is something remiss about our most cherished social program. Doctors, however, are not health economists, and just as you wouldn't want a health economist to remove your brain tumour, you wouldn't necessarily want a neurosurgeon to write a prescription for the overhaul of the health care system. That neurosurgeon may have some pretty good ideas, but wouldn't understand market forces, supply, and demand the way a trained health economist would. A two-tier health care system would not only be more expensive and prevent many from getting care, but it would not solve the accountability problems in the system.

This book is about accountability, mostly to the taxpayers who pay the bills. As owners of the system, we need to know what is being spent on medicare, and as patients we need information on the quality of doctors and hospitals.

Death and complication rates by doctor and by hospital are important measures of quality, as are the numbers of a specific operation a physician has done.

This book is not about bad news, nor is it a death-knell for our most cherished social program. It's a wake-up call for Canadians to become savvy consumers, for hospitals to push for higher standards, and for health care workers to treat all members of society equally and to do no harm, as the Hippocratic oath states. It is an attempt to arm Canadians with some tough questions to ask their doctors and hospitals, because information—and the publishing of it—will not only give patients true, informed consent, but it will help rid the system of inefficiencies and bad apples and make it competitive.

The real problem with medicare is that there is so little information. If we have guides to the best restaurants, hotels, and cars, why not a guide to the best hospitals for cancer care, orthopedics, dermatology, or obstetrics? Is it not reasonable to suggest that the very people paying into the system should at least know what they're purchasing? Our lives are on the line. But doctors and hospitals guard information with the excuse that it would be an invasion of privacy or, less convincingly, that the public wouldn't understand the information because it's too complex. In some cases, the information just isn't there, but that shouldn't be an excuse not to try to gather it.

"I think we have very little accountability," said former federal Health Minister Monique Bégin in an interview. "So little that, right now, the only channel of accountability would be a major, major health care crisis." It's for that reason that the topic of this book causes a certain amount of trepidation. Canadians justifiably want to hold on to the last social system that defines and connects them. There's nothing wrong and everything right with that, except when medicare is put on a pedestal. All the moral platitudes and boastfulness in the world can't keep a complex, multibillion health care system going. "There's a pathetic smugness that pervades our view of the health care system," said Kingston radiation oncologist Dr. William Mackillop, who has written on how the poor have far worse cancer survival rates than the rich. "But the only way to have a relatively good health care system is if people are prepared to be critical. It [the health care system] is weaker than it should be because people take an uncritical view of it."

In this book, you will learn that while new medical technologies are evaluated, the pairs of hands using them frequently aren't. That was particularly the case when keyhole gall-bladder surgery, medically known as laparoscopic cholecystectomy, was introduced in 1989 in Canada. Some doctors spent the weekend operating on pigs—sometimes in a hotel—and then moved straight to humans with varying results, while other hospitals were more diligent and made doctors perform a required number of operations under supervision before going solo on patients. As well, you will read about how some hospitals perform very low numbers of high-risk cancer surgeries, the things you cannot find out about your doctor, and how difficult it is to sue for malpractice once injured in a hospital. One cannot always control the outcome of medical treatment, but after reading this book and asking the right questions, you will be on the path to taking charge of your health care and lobbying for change.

Medicare must be operated on from the inside out. Experts can keep talking about ways to reform the health care system, but unless a sweeping series of adjustments in the form of accountability are made, it will all be for naught. Aggressive measures are going to have to be readied to make sure taxpayers and patients get the most bang for their health care buck.

Despite their collective investment, Canadians ask few questions and rarely demand returns on medicare. We feel that somehow we're getting health care for free, when actually we pay dearly through our taxes each year. Only when we know what we're spending our money on and know whether it works, can our health care system truly be on the road to recovery.

Like a marriage that's in need of restructuring, so too is medicare. While reforms are taking place across the country, the most important and contentious ingredient—quality control—is the least known component. The automobile industry couldn't survive not knowing if its cars worked, what they cost, and if they were safe to drive. Nor could the aviation industry. When a new plane is built, it goes through many inspections and the pilots receive very rigorous training and must meet spelled-out standards.

One thing is certain: What worked in the 1980s with

double-digit health budget increases doesn't work in the frugal 1990s. If hospitals have to reinvent themselves by dealing with fiscal restraints through more day surgeries and the desire for people to heal at home, then they're going to have to tell the public why that's important and give them something in the form of information.

There was a time, not too long ago, when hospitals that ran deficits were merely given more money by government, with few questions asked. They didn't have to show precisely what they were spending their money on, or whether it worked. It was as if those areas of health care were immeasurable and talking about their cost and effectiveness cheapened the notion of healing. "Hospitals have been strange institutions in that we couldn't tell you accurately about the cost of the product. We didn't have to—someone gave us a pot of money," said Ted Freedman, president of Mount Sinai Hospital in Toronto.

Although the fiscal restraints are on, medicare is not being made accountable to those it serves. For starters, here are a few questions that Canadians should be asking of their most favoured social program:

- **Should hospitals be rated?** Other countries are doing it, so why shouldn't Canada? All patients—not just those with "ins" in the medical community—deserve to know what hospital programs and physicians provide the best health care. Patients can then choose what they believe to be the best care, and hospitals would work to improve programs so they could be at the top of the list.

- **Which is more important, doctors' rights to privacy or patient safety?** Patients should know the complication rates, death rates, and readmission rates of procedures and operations by surgeons. "Scorecard medicine" might just ensure that doctors whose skills are slipping are tossed out or forced to shape up.

- **Are hospitals too soft on surgeons?** What should happen, for instance, if a hospital has an unacceptably high rate of gall-bladder removals, hysterectomies, or Caesarean sections? Whose job is it to make sure that fewer are performed? Right now, it's nobody's job.

- **Should we set "volume" standards on doctors performing surgeries, as the airline industry does on pilots?** The only thing arguably more dangerous than "high-volume" medicine, where doctors work to levels of excessive fatigue, is "low-volume" medicine, where physicians are doing so few of a procedure they are unable to keep their skills up. What should be done about this? Is lower-quality, accessible medicine preferred over first-rate care in a hospital that is an airplane ride away?

- **Should the sickest patients be treated the soonest?** Thousands and thousands of patients are on waiting lists in this country. With few exceptions, the sickest are not treated the quickest. Should that change and, if so, how?

- **Should it be easier for hospitals to terminate doctors whose skills are slipping?** When doctors are found to be practising substandard medicine, whose job is it to get rid of them or change their case loads so patients aren't harmed? Should there be a mandatory monitoring process for such doctors performed by an outside body? Are doctors' reputations being protected at the expense of the public?

As key shareholders in medicare, Canadians have a right to information on how their hospitals and doctors are performing. If the system is to stay solvent and improve, it's going to need the people who use it to speak out. Don't put off lobbying your politicians or asking the right questions until it's too late. Medicare's health—and your own—depends on being informed.

## *One*

# Tragedy by the Dozen

*Winnipeg*—Just a few more hours and everything will be better. Or at least that's what Ben Capili thought that September 13, 1994, as he waited for his daughter Marietess to roll out of the operating room doors at Health Sciences Centre (HSC). He imagined smiling doctors pulling off their surgical masks, shaking his hand and assuring him Marietess was going to be fine after having congenital heart defects repaired. But he couldn't shake this anxious feeling. Was this the normal worry of a parent? Or had something gone wrong? Then he remembered the words of the surgeon who had told him the operation would be a "walk in the park." Feeling a little more settled, twenty-three-year-old Capili sat in the waiting room and quietly waited for word.

Capili's thoughts wandered to the night before when he and Sarah Tena, Marietess's mother, had had an argument in the hospital corridor. He couldn't recall what the quarrel was about—probably something petty—but he did remember feeling bruised about it. Marietess had interrupted the dispute, exclaiming, "I love you, Dad." His heart had swelled. Just a few hours before that quarrel, they had explained to Marietess as best as parents can that her heart was going to be fixed. "We promise you, your heart will be better," Capili recalled saying. "They're going to put you to sleep and then fix your heart," he had told his daughter, months away from her third birthday.

Just after 4 p.m., a nurse approached Capili and Tena in the waiting room. "They're just finishing up," she told them. "Everything is going as planned." They felt relieved. An hour later, pediatric cardiac surgeon Dr. Jonah Odim came out and said the operation went well. "When you see her, she'll be pink. There are a few minor problems with a blood clot," Capili recalled Odim saying.

It wasn't until 8 p.m. that Marietess was rolled out of the operating room and into the pediatric intensive care unit, but the sight of her was anything but rosy. "Her head was four times the [normal] size and blue. It was grotesque," Capili recalled. Something was definitely wrong. "Why does she look that way?" Capili asked. It was suggested to him that after heart surgery babies "usually look like this." Capili hesitantly accepted this explanation and left shortly after, wanting to believe all was well. A nurse would later remark that Marietess's head had really looked like a "big grape."

A telephone ringing in the middle of the night awoke Capili. "Marietess isn't doing too well," the voice on the other end of the phone said. Capili threw on his clothes in a panic and rushed down to HSC, an 860-bed hospital that stretches through 79 hectares of downtown Winnipeg. When he arrived, he was told that Marietess would probably not recover. About a half hour later, Marietess died. Just like that. Odim mentioned something to him about fluid around the lungs, but Capili didn't understand what that meant. All he could think was, "My little girl is dead." As Capili walked into Marietess's room, he noticed a very spotless floor and a bloated, purplish child lying on crisp hospital sheets. Marietess seemed so foreign to him, her beautiful features barely recognizable in the middle of the sterile hospital room. "All I could remember is that her head was bloated, there were bruises everywhere, and everything was so damn clean."

That day, and for many days after it, Capili would try to find out what had gone wrong. But doctors and other hospital officials would not be immediately forthcoming.

What Capili could not have known is that Marietess was the first patient operated on by Odim following a summer moratorium on high-risk pediatric cardiac surgery. But the Winnipeg pediatric cardiac program had had troubles before then. It was first shut down in 1983, restarted in 1986, discontinued in 1993, then started up again in 1994. There was a brief moratorium that year, then it was restarted—only to be indefinitely suspended in 1995.

If Capili had learned that the unit had been closed, he would have had the option of sending his child elsewhere—

such as to Saskatoon or Toronto—and possibly changing the course of fate. "If they had told me it had closed down, we would have gone—right off the bat. Once you heard the program has shut down, you wouldn't want anything to do with it."

Capili also didn't know anything about Odim's credentials, how long he had been a surgeon, or how many operations of this type he had done previously unassisted. Nor did Capili know how long the operating team had been together or how the Winnipeg pediatric cardiac program rated compared to similar programs in Canada. Even if, under all the stress of having a sick child, he had thought to ask these questions, he likely wouldn't have received many answers.

Marietess's death left her parents devastated. That and a number of other things caused them to separate. "My rights as a parent to do the best for my child were taken away from me," said Capili. He decided to put his job as a gas station attendant on hold for one year to devote himself to learning the truth about Marietess's death. He began by calling nurses, hospital officials, Dr. Odim, and cardiologist Dr. Niels Giddins. On more than one occasion, a receptionist told Capili that the doctors were "very busy." After four months Capili hadn't had as much as an appointment with doctors, nor had he been able to obtain a copy of his daughter's final autopsy report.

Then, as Capili was driving his car that winter, he heard a snippet on the radio, something about the infant heart surgery unit being indefinitely suspended at HSC. The pediatric heart unit was closed, ironically, on Valentine's Day, 1995. He knew it—something *was* definitely going on. He raced home, telephoned the hospital, demanded a copy of Marietess's final autopsy report, and asked for a meeting with the doctors involved. Capili finally got his meeting with Odim and Giddins but, although the meeting lasted more than four hours, he received little useful information. He did remember Giddins being somewhat dismissive, saying, "You can't believe everything you read in the papers."

Shortly after that blurb on the radio, Capili called Manitoba NDP health critic Dave Chomiak, who was keeping in touch with reporters at the *Winnipeg Free Press*. Chomiak was fielding calls at his North Kildonan constituency office and at the Manitoba Legislature from distraught parents who were unsatisfied with explanations of how their babies died. "Parents were clearly not informed adequately," Chomiak said. "They were being danced around, played around with—they were being victimized."

Parents were now banding together and asking tough questions of the hospital and the medical establishment, and demanding an inquiry into the deaths of their children. Not long after, chief medical examiner Dr. Peter Markesteyn called an inquest into the dozen babies who had died under the new surgical program headed by Dr. Odim, a young physician with a brilliant curriculum vitae and a knack for scientific research.

Appointed to head the inquest was Associate Chief Justice Murray Sinclair, a well-liked man with a reputation for doing what is fair. Initially, parents were angry—they wanted a full-scale inquiry—and some even walked out of a February 1995 meeting with Crown attorneys Don Slough and Christina Kopynsky. "As far as we're concerned, the inquest is over," said Ron Fincaryk, whose son, Colt Unger-Fincaryk, died in 1989. "The taxpayers will pay a lot of money for it but that's all that's going to happen," he was quoted as saying in a *Winnipeg Free Press* newspaper story under the headline "Inquest a sham: parents." Margaret Feakes, a grandmother of one of the twelve babies, said Sinclair's appointment was the only positive development in the case.

Once parents got used to the idea that Sinclair would run the inquest, they became more comfortable. Sinclair, who had traded in his trade-mark, waist-length, thick braid for an off-the-shoulder ponytail, had a reputation for getting to the bottom of things. In the late 1980s, he co-chaired the Aboriginal Justice Inquiry after the murder of Helen Betty Osborne, a Cree high school student, went unsolved for sixteen years and a native leader was shot dead by police on a Winnipeg street. Quietly intelligent, Sinclair was as eager to learn the truth as many of the parents.

The inquest began in March 1996 and parents, relatives, and members of the public packed into the fourth floor Broadway Avenue courtroom. So, too, did lawyers—as many as ten at a time—representing the anesthetists, surgeons, cardiologists, and perfusionists (technicians who specialize in running the heart-lung bypass machines). Lawyers' fees for doctors are paid by the Canadian Medical Protective Association (CMPA), the physicians' malpractice insurance body, which is largely subsidized by taxpayers. The remainder is paid for by the doctors.

Parents of patients also received assistance. After lobbying the Manitoba government, parents received $25,000 per family to be represented at the inquest. Lawyers later obtained another $50,000 each from the province. Although some have complained the money was inadequate, five of the seven sets of parents suing pooled their funds and had lawyer Saul Simmonds represent them. As Simmonds noted, "None of these people can afford to sue anybody. How does the little person sue a doctor?" Eventually, two sets of parents dropped their suits.

Simmonds told parents that a successful malpractice suit for a dead infant would garner them anywhere from $10,000 to $30,000. That is dramatically different from the United States, where multimillion dollar settlements make the headlines. "Unfortunately, the death of a child in Canada is worth very, very small amounts of money," said Simmonds, himself the father of a young son. But the money wasn't of interest to many of the parents; they sued mostly because it was their last chance for justice.

Eventually, the inquest's scope broadened to look not only at twelve deaths out of forty-four children operated on by Odim in 1994, but at eighty-eight other children who died between 1981 and 1993 in the pediatric cardiac program. Sinclair and others spent their days poring through evidence, tens of thousands of pages of testimony, confidential memos, and dozens of reports as they tried to isolate the most important issues.

Although many wanted to blame Odim, there were other worrisome issues that extended beyond his scalpel. A Toronto Sick Children's Hospital team was convinced that more than surgical competence was at issue. Previous reports suggested that Manitoba may not have had the population to sustain a pediatric cardiac program. There may not have been enough patients for a surgeon and other members of the operating room team to maintain their skills. Unlike in some U.S. states, Canadian hospitals do not have to apply for a "certificate of need" to prove that a proposed program would have the required volume of surgeries needed for surgeons to maintain their skills. Also, there was no plan to take on less risky cases before gradually moving to the riskier ones, and a young, newly-trained surgeon did not have anyone to guide him and help him shoulder this awesome responsibility. To add to that, it didn't appear that the hospital conducted any extensive assessment of Odim's surgical skills before signing him on—a practice that is not unusual in Canada.

Dr. Bob Blanchard, head of surgery at HSC during the time of the deaths, testified that it was "a serious error on my part" to allow Dr. Odim to perform cardiac surgery on children without any support from a "senior mentor or team-builder." In a letter to Toronto's Hospital for Sick Children doctors, which was entered into evidence, Blanchard wrote: "Unfortunately we left Jonah [Odim] to fend for himself in a new environment with different procedures than he had previously experienced. He did not know our team and our team did not know him."

The biggest problem for most of the parents was that they could not get any information on what went wrong in the operating room. Not during the surgery, nor after their children died. "No one was talking to the parents. Even when serious problems seemed to occur, they were really kept in the dark," said Simmonds. "No one said, 'We're dealing with a new surgeon. Here's a guy with a great deal of academic experience and who looks wonderful on paper. The hospital has an obligation to assess him.'"

And "wonderful" isn't too strong a word. Odim's résumé included a medical degree from Yale University in 1981, followed by an internship and residency at the University of Chicago until 1987. He was appointed a fellow in cardiovascular and thoracic surgery at McGill University from 1987 to 1992, which included training in experimental surgery at Montreal General with Dr. Ray Chui. He finished training in 1993 with Dr. Aldo Castenada, who is reputed to be a leading pediatric heart surgeon in North America.

In an attempt to lure Dr. Odim to Winnipeg, HSC doctors Dr. Helmut Unruh, acting head of cardiothoracic surgery, and cardiologist Dr. George Collins did the usual wining and dining reserved for the medical establishment. "I thought that this was a confident, self-assured, and respectful young man who I thought I could work with very well. And I had some reason to believe that he had good surgical credentials," Collins would later testify. But he did notice that Odim was a bit more formal than most doctors. "He behaves in very much the way I would expect a mature young consultant to behave in that British system. But it's a little more formal than we are used to in the Canadian system."

On November 9, 1993, Blanchard offered the posting to Odim, who would receive unspecified fees for his services, including a $50,000 salary to cover the university portion of the appointment. In a letter written in September, Odim had asked Blanchard for a salary "in the range of $250,000 to $275,000 Cdn"—plus expenses. The contract to hire Odim guaranteed him $255,000 a year, no matter how many surgeries he performed.

The newly trained surgeon from Boston set up HSC's pediatric cardiac program in February 1994, after completing his training a year earlier. Although Winnipeg isn't exactly Boston, with its ivy-league universities and its large number of pediatric heart operations, the program was a prestigious one and could allow Odim to make his mark. HSC, too, must have been pleased to restart its program, especially since it was precisely the kind it needed to help maintain its teaching status and show the medical world it was a serious hospital.

When Odim arrived at HSC in the dead of winter, he must have experienced culture shock. Odim, an African-American, found himself living in a city with a large Ukrainian population. Winnipeg is also frightfully cold, with temperatures dropping to 40 degrees below zero in the winter. Smack in the middle of Canada and isolated, the city of 667,000 people makes up for its gruelling cold winters with its share of good theatre, funky nightspots, hot summers, and homes that are among the most reasonably priced in the country. Some joke that Winnipeg has two seasons—ten months of winter and two months of bad skiing—when, in fact, it has some of the prettiest beaches in the country a short drive north of the city.

When Odim arrived at HSC, operating room nurse Carol Youngson attempted to schedule a meeting with him. She assumed he would want to meet with her and some other members of the operating team to discuss instruments, sutures, and the like. There was the suggestion of doing a dry run, since Odim was new and the pediatric cardiac program had been defunct for several months. That way, they could show how the lines from the pump were positioned and help to ensure the first cases went smoothly. But the dry run never took place.

Days later the operations began, and Youngson felt Odim was having some trouble with what is medically referred to as cannulation, a procedure where the patient is put onto a heart-lung machine that artificially circulates blood during surgery. To Youngson, he initially seemed almost unfamiliar with the procedure. It didn't take long before Odim felt that he was having some difficulty establishing himself as captain of the ship and that his hands were almost tied. He also noted that there was a "lack of local leadership in cardiac surgery, cardiology, and anesthesia."

Early on in the program, some babies encountered trouble in the intensive care unit shortly after surgery, and some had to be rushed back to the OR to have their chests reopened. But in pediatric cardiac surgery it isn't just the cutting and sewing that determines if a child lives or dies.

"The surgery is often just the first of two or three major hurdles that you have to get over. The second is getting off the ventilator and the third one is getting to be able to feed and begin to grow," said pediatric cardiac surgeon Dr. Kim Duncan, who operated on babies before Dr. Odim took over the program. Pediatric cardiac surgery is probably some of the most difficult surgery around. "Without any question, of all the surgery that I have seen, pediatric cardiac surgery is the most complex," HSC cardiac surgeon Dr. George Hamilton would later testify. "Half the time the diagnosis is not quite what you thought it was when you get in there, and you see these little egg-beater hearts that are all stirred up, and you have got to figure out where the red blood goes, and it is all time-dependent. You have to think in 3-D, while the clock is ticking." As well, surgeons are "working on a thing the size of an acorn. I mean, you see a neonatal heart, these things aren't big," said Hamilton, who was later ordered by senior hospital officials to assist Odim with all high-risk and newborn heart surgeries.

Only a few weeks into the program, nine-month-old Gary Caribou died after a patching of a hole in the heart turned into a lengthy surgery. Gary had been diagnosed with a hole in his heart two months earlier by a cardiologist, but instead of being referred elsewhere for surgery, he was sent back home to Lynn Lake, more than 1000 kilometres north of Winnipeg, where he was hooked up to feeding tubes in the local hospital. Gary's mother, Charlotte Caribou, was told her son's heart condition required surgery, "the sooner the better."

After waiting two months, with no explanation for the delay, Gary was returned to Winnipeg for surgery on March 14, 1994, but there were difficulties during the operation, the biggest of which was that surgeons could not close his chest because his heart was too swollen. Instead, they covered Gary with a piece of material. Caribou asked to hold her son. Nestled in his mother's arms, the boy—wrapped in a white hospital blanket—looked almost as if he was sleeping. When Caribou asked doctors what had happened, she was told the operation took nine hours because "they couldn't find the hole in his heart because there was more muscle [around the heart] than they thought." (The doctors eventually found and patched the hole.)

Caribou would later hear that Gary had what is medically known as ventricle septal defects, or holes in the pumping portion of his heart. Caribou was told that only between eight and twelve cases out of a hundred run into difficulty during Gary's type of operation. Although Odim had performed the operation unassisted only once six years earlier in Montreal, he didn't feel the inexperience elevated the risk. "I felt confident. It wasn't an issue," he testified.

Surgery continued in Operating Room 2 under the eleven-member team, and so did the deaths. The second to join the roster of the dead was eight-month-old Jessica Ulimaumi, of Arviat, NWT, who died on March 27, 1994, after a tube that connected her to a bypass machine in the intensive care unit fell out. Essentially, she bled to death when a critical hose pumping her blood into a heart-lung machine was inadvertently left unclamped. During an autopsy, a needle was found lodged in a major blood vessel. Although Jessica's death did not occur in the operating room, "the cause was likely related to surgical technique," said a report later penned by the pediatric death review committee of Manitoba's College of Physicians and Surgeons, the doctors' regulatory body. The committee did not name Jessica and three other children but described their surgeries, making it easy to identify them.

Later, Odim would blame his assisting surgeon for not clamping the line connecting Jessica to the heart bypass machine, but he conceded that he was in charge and that he should have recognized that the clamp wasn't put on. Before Jessica was wheeled out of the operating room following eight hours of surgery, nurses noted a needle was missing but no X-ray was done to find out if it had been left in her chest, as hospital policy required.

Four-year-old Vinay Goyal was the next to die after undergoing a second operation to repair a hole in his heart, as the first operation did not completely close it. He died on the operating room table from massive bleeding. Though they identified Vinay by case and not by name, the college's pediatric death review committee concluded the boy's demise was "possibly preventable with improved medical management."

The parents of these children were not lax. They asked questions, and tried to get the best possible care for their children. Danica and Karl Terziski, parents of Daniel, even offered to fly in Dr. Christo Tchervenkov, director of cardiovascular surgery at Montreal Children's Hospital, at their own expense to help Dr. Odim operate on their son. "We thought two heads were better than one," Danica Terziski said. But Giddins apparently was opposed to recruiting help for Odim, who had started his surgical job only six weeks before.

The Terziskis tried to figure out the best course of action for their son, who needed a high-risk Norwood operation. (A Norwood is a series of three complex reconstructive surgeries that involves patching a hole in the heart and switching the placement of the pulmonary and aortic arteries, which allows the heart to pump blood normally.) The couple said they received many conflicting opinions. First, Danica Terziski was told by Odim that the Norwood procedure was performed in centres such as Boston, Montreal, and Toronto, but Giddins told her that Odim had worked with the world's best surgeons and Winnipeg had a team capable of performing the surgery. She pressed Odim again for his opinion on which centre was the best place to have the surgery. "I asked him, 'If this was your child, where would you have the surgery?' He said, 'It's not my child. It's not my place to comment,'" Terziski testified.

Daniel died on April 20, 1994, after undergoing the Norwood operation. The Terziskis were given fifty-fifty odds that the surgery would work, but in retrospect those figures were extremely generous. A report by Toronto's Hospital for Sick Children entered into evidence found the real death rate from Norwoods and the arterial switch operation was more like eighty to one hundred per cent.

The Terziskis did everything they possibly could to obtain

the best outcome for their child, but still it wasn't enough. Arguably, a lack of essential information meant they were not able to shop around properly for surgical care. Thinking back, Danica Terziski wonders what might have happened had she been given more information. "Maybe my child might still be alive if I had been better informed," she said outside the courtroom after testifying. "If [only] there was a better business bureau of doctors to say whether this one is better or more capable than that one [at a certain procedure]."

The tally of the dead was growing, just ten weeks into the program, with five out of fourteen babies operated on passing away, including Alyssa Still, who had surgery on May 4, 1994, came out of it alive, but then died two days later.

Also at death's door was the morale in the operating room. By May 19, 1994—only a few months after the program had begun—a core team of cardiac nurses met to discuss their concerns. They felt it was "very demoralizing to lose so many patients in so short a time," according to nurses' notes entered into evidence.

One of the nurses, Carol Youngson, testified that she had asked the head of pediatric surgery, Dr. Nathan Wiseman, for help "several times throughout the year. I pleaded with him to just come in and see what was going on. I needed reassurance I wasn't going crazy." But she said Wiseman refused to watch Odim work, saying, "No, I can't do that." Youngson, a veteran with 23 years of experience in operating rooms working with more than 150 surgeons, felt haunted by what she felt were needless deaths caused by "something we were doing in the operative field." She had to restrain herself from warning parents to go away. "If I had gone to this parent and said, 'Stop. You can't do this. Take your baby and run,'" she said at the inquest, "all hell would have broken loose. I would have looked like an over-emotional, almost crazy person."

The nurses weren't the only ones taking action. Anesthetists threatened to boycott any further surgeries by Odim and requested a review of the patients operated on. In a memo to Wiseman, the members of pediatric anesthesia "unanimously agreed that pending the recommendations of the immediate review we suspend the provision of cardiac anesthesia for open cases as of Tuesday, May 17, 1994."

Dr. Ann McNeill was one of the concerned anesthetists. "Over fifty per cent of the children under a year who had bypass died," she testified later at the inquest. "I think that when we decided that we wanted to, that we had to, raise our concerns. Rightly or wrongly we met with a reaction which surprised us at the time from many corners. There were people who were with us and supported us, but there were also people who were outraged at what we had done and the manner in which we had done it."

Since doctors rarely react rashly to their colleagues, this move by anesthetists was a rather extraordinary one. As anesthetist Dr. Harley Wong later testified, "As you all know, for one doctor to make a formal complaint against another is extraordinary. The traditional relationship between surgeon and anesthetist makes the stance we took in May 1994 even more extraordinary."

Dr. Douglas Craig, head of HSC's anesthesia department, apparently didn't take kindly to the move and told anesthetists that if they had staged a similar revolt in the United States, they'd be out of jobs, McNeill testified. "He was angry with us, at what he perceived to be obstructive, negative, critical protests against high-risk surgery," she said. Other tactics to get the four anesthetists to stop their job action included a warning by their immediate supervisor and suggestions that they could be replaced.

According to Wong, anesthetists were thrust into a "no-win situation." First, their opinions obviously were not taken very seriously and if they said something to patients, they worried they would be accused of undermining the hospital. Then there was the problem of patients. Did they have a duty to tell them of the deaths? "Because we did not say anything to the parents then our ethics are also being questioned," Wong testified. Still, he wanted to know how much he should inform patients. "If I know that surgeon A has a higher mortality and morbidity rate for surgery X than surgeon B, then what is my obligation to that patient?" he asked Sinclair.

Despite the nurses' and the anesthetists' action and a quality control system at HSC that routinely monitors patient care and "medication errors," top-ranking hospital executives said they were not informed of the operating-room problems in the unit until December 1994.

The anesthetists' May 1994 boycott eventually did get the attention of some hospital officials, who called a crisis meeting. The anesthetists relented and agreed to work with

Odim on low-risk cases. The hospital also created a special committee headed by Wiseman. The so-called Wiseman committee was to steer the pediatric cardiac program "in a manner which is agreeable to all involved individuals," according to a hospital memo. That spring, committee members decided to temporarily defer patients who were of a "more complex/high-risk nature." No reason was given in the internal hospital memo for this move, other than the fact that "it was generally felt that this would be the best course to pursue during the review period." The committee held several more meetings and at one of them in the fall of that year, mentioned that eleven babies had been sent out of province to Saskatoon, Edmonton and Toronto over a period of three months.

Meanwhile, two babies died between May and September. Shalynn Piller was given a ninety-two per cent chance of successful surgery to repair a narrow aorta, and although the surgery seemed to work, the baby's condition deteriorated afterward and the fourteen-day-old died on August 4 in what at the time her mother said was "God's will." Eight-month-old Aric Baumann was born with a small hole between the left and right ventricles and although the operation closed the hole, Aric could not be weaned off the respirator and died on August 21, two months after surgery.

In late August, the Wiseman Committee noted there was "significant pressure" to increase the number of operations according to committee minutes. In early September, it would recommend the program be fully reactivated, which it was.

One month later in October, Giddins informed the committee that two high-risk procedures had been successfully performed by Odim: one on a child with Down's syndrome, and the other on a child who had had a bilateral shunt. A shunt sends more blood into the lungs by connecting a vessel from the main artery, the aorta, to the lungs. Certainly this was good news, and some took it as a sign that things were improving.

But it didn't take long for the tension to build among the operating room staff. The eleven-member team worked in a small room, squeezed in, careful not to trip over the dozens of wires and cords on the floor. Perfusionists, technicians who specialize in running the heart-lung bypass machines, were also finding it difficult to work with Odim. "I tried to remain professional and go when I was scheduled," testified Todd Koga later. But Koga admitted that pediatric cardiac surgery with this team was "starting to lose its glow."

It was also starting to lose more babies. One nurse testified that some parents of ailing infants—particularly those with medical connections or middle-class or affluent backgrounds—sent their babies out of Manitoba to institutions such as Toronto's Hospital for Sick Children, which is world-renowned. HSC nurse Irene Hinam would later testify that doctors and nurses went so far as to advise friends and relatives to take their babies away, but aboriginal and lower middle-class families were not extended any such alternative.

Hinam later testified, "I said, 'One of these days this is not going to be an aboriginal child [who dies]. This is not going to be a child from up north. It is going to be an upper middle-class white family that has the ins [connections] into the medical system and is going to know that this shouldn't have happened. And there is going to be a lawsuit.'"

Sadly, nurses who once loved looking after these sick infants now dreaded entering the unit. "Staff attitudes towards caring for the post-op[erative] cardiac patient have changed dramatically," nurses wrote in a memo. "Previously, all staff looked forward to cardiac admissions and caring for these children. Now no one will volunteer and staff verbally state they do not want to care for these children." This wasn't just the feeling of the less-experienced nurses; it was felt even by those who had more than a decade of experience. In fact, "nurses with more than ten years of previous PICU [pediatric intensive care unit] experience state that they feel physically ill on thinking of coming to work when there is a fresh cardiac patient." Many nurses said openly that they would not allow a family member or friend with a heart lesion to have surgery at HSC. When asked why, their responses included: "It's so depressing." "I don't know what to say to families." "Before, we used to know what to expect." But that changed as "even the simplest cases do so poorly." "I feel we are deceiving the parents."

For his part, Odim knew there were personality conflicts, but he didn't realize how deeply they ran. "Certainly in 1994 I wasn't aware of how deep some of those problems were with certain individuals. Certainly with some of them in the OR like Ms. Youngson, there clearly was, you know, some difficulty, but I did not appreciate the severity of it until much later, when the program had been shut down," he later testified.

Odim also told the reviewers from the Toronto Hospital for Sick Children that after he arrived, he felt that there was no leadership for the anesthetists and that support staff failed to respond to his requests. In addition, he claimed that there was no process to address problems and that he had little support from the hospital. Odim said he preferred to practise surgery the way he was trained, favouring "a complete definitive repair" on sick babies, rather than the less complex operations previously performed in the program. Odim felt he "was being made the problem" as he went from being "as good as, if not better than, the previous surgeon," to being a scapegoat.

Hamilton, a cardiac surgeon, heard rumblings about anesthetists' concerns around the same time he noticed Odim was becoming "quieter and withdrawn a little bit. And I think that he was … getting depressed." Although Hamilton thought his colleague's "skills were certainly adequate to do the job," he felt Odim was rather unseasoned and thrown "into the deep end of the water." But Hamilton thought it unfortunate that his colleague "didn't put the brakes on things."

Once babies made it out of intensive care, they still weren't out of the woods. Nurses said a "significant number of these children go on to require permanent pacemakers; previously this was a rare occurrence." There was also "notable increase" in bleeding following the operations. "If no problems arose, they could manage. However,

Dr. Odim seemed to be unprepared for problems as they occurred and was often without a plan for action." Youngson wrote she witnessed "several instances of sloppy and careless surgical technique," while others voiced their concerns about Odim's skill and "hurried approach to his work. While we realize that time is of the essence ... it is our opinion that on many occasions Dr. Odim, in an effort to be fast, sacrificed good surgical technique and judgement at the expense of the patient," said Youngson's notes.

Over the next few months, the roster of the deceased grew with the deaths of Capili's daughter Marietess, Erica Bichel, Ashton Feakes, Jesse Maguire, and Erin Petkau. Although the parents of these children were given varying explanations for their babies' deaths, none of them was made aware of the program's troubled history.

Laurie Maguire was one mother who was suspicious when her son died. Sensing something was wrong, she insisted on seeing the autopsy report, which stated that a "tear" had occurred. In a meeting she arranged with Dr. Odim and Dr. Cameron Ward, who has since taken a job in Australia, Maguire said the pair focused on two lengthy periods when Jesse was on an artificial heart-lung machine. They also noted an obstruction in the baby's blood vessel. "They were nervous. Dr. Odim in particular. He looked really nervous," Maguire told the inquest. Even though the temperature of the meeting room was cool, she said the doctors were sweating that day. Ward, whom Maguire described as a "warm" physician, was the more nervous of the two. "I got the impression he felt something was wrong

... he was crying. You had to see the look on his face. It was incredible. It was as bad as mine."

Although Maguire was told her two-day-old son died because he could not come off the pump machine, that was only part of the problem. There was chaos in the operating room on November 27, 1994, when the aorta cannula was dislodged and fell out, according to nurses' notes entered into evidence at the inquest, but it wasn't until that inquest that Maguire said she found out about it. "During the rewarming process the aortic cannula was dislodged and fell out. Both the surgeon and the assistant (Dr. Hancock) struggled for six or seven minutes to replace the cannula. They were very disorganized and panicky," the nurses' notes said. "They argued with each other and grabbed the cannula and instruments from one another and it was very obvious that NEITHER ONE HAD THE SKILL OR EXPERTISE TO HANDLE THIS SITUATION," said the notes (their emphasis).

Odim was "extremely rough, 'jamming' the cannula in again and again ... . It was noted that the surgical field was extremely messy and unorganized throughout the case." After the aortic tear was noticed, Odim "remarked to the anesthetist at the end of the case that he should have been much more meticulous with his cannulation technique." According to the nurses' notes, "it was discovered that the aortic repair was destroyed as well as a tear in the posterior (back) wall of the aorta ... . The baby died in the OR. Dr. Odim ... discussed with the cardiologist (in front of several people in the OR) what the parents of this child should be told. It was decided not to tell them about the problems with the cannula—only that they were unable to come off the pump."

Perfusionist Michael Maas would later describe it as a "catastrophic event." Even if Jesse had survived surgery, Maas testified that there were risks of brain damage because he had spent two hours and forty-nine minutes in total circulatory arrest. That was the time it took to do the operation and to repair the torn aorta. As Crown attorney Don Slough pointed out during the inquest, the amount of time Jesse Maguire was on the heart pump was "off the scale."

When Maguire heard about the tear, "I thought: 'You bunch of liars.' That's how I felt," she testified. For his part, Odim testified that he told Maguire the whole story. It probably didn't help Maguire that a Manitoba College of Physicians and Surgeons report concluded that her son's death was related to surgical technique. "There is a need for a timely, accountable, concurrent audit process at the hospital level whenever complex multi-disciplinary programs of this nature are undertaken on children," concluded the report by the college's pediatric death review committee. In all, the committee noted four deaths (Capili, Goyal, Ulimaumi, and Maguire) as being "possibly preventable with improved medical management." In two of the cases, Ulimaumi and Maguire, the deaths were also related to surgical technique.

Later, Maguire told a newspaper reporter that "until you lose a child, you will never know how much it hurts.

It is incredible pain that I carry with me every day. It never goes away. I wanted to die right along with Jesse. The only thing that kept me going was that I was born Catholic and they say if you take your own life you won't go to heaven and I didn't want to risk never seeing Jesse again." During her testimony, Maguire stressed to Sinclair that he should recommend against high-risk, open-heart surgery being done on children in Manitoba unless there is proper staffing and equipment. "These are not guinea pigs. These are children they're working on."

Other parents crumbled on the witness stand as they attempted to cope with their grief. Some brought photographs of their deceased children to show Sinclair. One woman, Charlotte Caribou, travelled all night by bus from Lynn Lake, 1079 kilometres north of Winnipeg, to testify at the inquest.

Meanwhile, headlines in the *Winnipeg Free Press* couldn't have been any more descriptive. "Kids Lucky to be Alive;" "Nightmare in Manitoba: Nurse;" "Parents Kept in the Dark: Nurse."

Eventually, the inquest turned its attention to the death of Marietess Capili, who was rolled into Operating Room 2 on September 13, 1994. There was trouble even before the operation began. Marietess was lying on the operating room table, with tubes coming out of her body and her head out of view, which is typical in operations. A piece of cloth was draped over her neck so that the only person who would see her head on a regular basis would be the anesthetist, who stood and sat at the head of the table, watching the levels of oxygen, blood gases, and blood pressure machines among other things.

Odim apparently had difficulty getting Marietess onto the heart-lung machine, which artificially circulates blood during surgery—a procedure medically known as cannulation. An operating room nurse noted that Odim did the procedure "with great difficulty and [at] risk to [the] patient." The first cannula—or intravenous line—used on Marietess was too big. "This was pointed out to the surgeon. He tried to insert it and this resulted in a tear in the vessel," according to nurses' notes. Marietess then became unstable. After Odim put the three cannulae in place, Marietess had to go onto the heart pump quickly because of her unstable vital signs.

The operative field was "very disorganized," and while trying to go on bypass a clamp was unwittingly left on the venous line of Marietess. That means that a clamp was left on the superior vena cava, a blood vessel which brings blood from the head and upper body back to the heart. The perfusionist told Odim there was "no flow," but it was the circulating nurse who finally noticed it by looking at the baby's head which was behind a cloth, out of the surgeon's sight. Nurses suspected the young patient was suffering from superior vena cava syndrome, which was causing Marietess's head to balloon with blood that had no way to return to her heart. Also, a post-mortem found that a suture from surgery had narrowed the right superior vena cava and the anomalous left superior vena cava.

Nurses, doctors, and other members of the operating

room relayed more stories of what occurred in Operating Room 2. Problems with the surgeries and communication, and no one person in charge, were the recurrent messages at the inquest. Some nurses and doctors also wondered aloud if parents of patients should have been given more information before consenting to the operations. Neonatal intensive care unit nurses wrote that a "more honest approach needs to be taken regarding outcomes." In the end, it was the neonatologists, doctors who specialize in looking after newborns, who had the greatest impact when they refused to accept pediatric cardiac patients. That made it virtually impossible for Odim and his team to continue, as they had no patients to operate on.

Giddins, too, testified to having "concerns" about the program and intended to speak to Dr. Brian Postl, head of pediatrics and child health. However, the program was closed before he had a chance, he testified. As the only cardiologist left out of four on staff, Giddins said he was plunged into a fiscal-medical maelstrom with no authority over developments. "It was a pervasively, bizarrely, stressful existence," he testified, adding that he was often on call twenty-four hours a day.

Odim performed his final surgery on December 22, 1994, and left for Christmas vacation a day later. HSC then hired two Hospital for Sick Children doctors to evaluate the beleaguered program. Drs. Bill Williams and W.L. Roy flew to Winnipeg and spent two days there in late January, interviewing those involved in the program. Their days began at 7:30 in the morning and went through until early evening, while they talked to nurses, anesthetists, pediatric surgeons, and others. They also pored over hospital statistics. Their sixteen-page report was sent to Dr. R.J.W. Blanchard, chair of the department of surgery for the University of Manitoba.

Perhaps not surprisingly, the report answered some of the darkest fears of HSC staff. Yes, the death rates for the program were "unacceptable." The twenty-nine per cent death rate for babies under one year old was far in excess of the eleven per cent at Toronto's Hospital for Sick Children, which operates on some of the most complex baby cases in Canada. (The death rate was also higher than in the program's previous six years.) Bypass times and aortic cross-clamp times were "excessive and much longer than a random sample generated from the Hospital for Sick Children, Toronto," Williams and Roy wrote. In some cases, the prolonged times were attributable to the "learning curve of a new and junior pediatric surgeon." However, the "reviewers are convinced that more than surgical competence is at issue and other important deficiencies must be corrected before resuming pediatric cardiac surgery." They also paraphrased a HSC neonatologist when they noted that no cardiovascular surgery program is preferable to a program with unacceptable complication and death rates. Forty-two neonates with cardiac disease had been airlifted to other centres without significant complications, they pointed out.

Williams and Roy also made a few other observations. First, it would be very difficult for pediatric cardiac anesthetists to maintain their skills due to the small number of cases. Second, although some charged that the anesthetists were not committed to the program, the reviewers felt they were probably "very committed at the outset but this commitment has been eroded over the ten-month period" and "these degenerating relations (between the surgeon and members of the cardiac anaesthesia team) may affect patient care."

They recommended that neonatal patients with complex lesions be transferred to a larger, more experienced centre, as "the small referral base for this program (one million) may ultimately preclude any effort to develop increased experience in managing these complex lesions." In retrospect, the reviewers felt that "these patients and the program might have benefited from a more gradual introduction of cases."

Even though the reviewers did not observe Odim in the operating theatre, they felt there was "evidence to at least question the technical competence of the present cardiovascular surgeon." Although complex cases, unfamiliar equipment, and support staff produced a recipe for the program's "derailment," the situation was further compounded by a lack of diplomacy on the part of a new, young surgeon who may have been judged unfairly by some of his colleagues. "One observer stated 'he [Odim] was the last to advise but the first to criticize,'" when in fact, "the real problem was [Odim's] frustration arising from negative results, absence of institutional support, and unreasonably high expectations." They also found that the program was poorly supported by the institution from the outset, and that a "serious crisis of confidence" existed between the cardiac surgeon and the anesthetists and "virtually all nurses attached to the cardiac program."

One option suggested by the reviewers was to combine the Manitoba and Saskatchewan surgical units so there would be "an appropriate critical mass [number] of children with congenital heart disease." Recent studies comparing sizes of various pediatric units in United States hospitals found that larger units are not only more cost effective, but have better survival rates and fewer complications. In 1994, when Odim was there, HSC's unit performed eighty procedures—some of them highly complex—which some have suggested could be too low a number for some members of the operating room team to maintain excellence.

Ten days after receiving the report, HSC president Rod Thorfinnson, his senior staff, and two senior Health Department officials met to discuss it. Then Deputy Health Minister Dr. John Wade, who is also an anesthetist by training, and Assistant Deputy Minister Tim Duprey were included as observers. Wade spoke of his long-standing concern that the population of Manitoba was just too small to sustain a viable pediatric cardiac surgery program. By that, he meant that there may not have been enough ill babies for surgeons to operate on to keep their skills up. It was at this meeting that HSC officials said they discussed officially suspending the program indefinitely.

On Monday, February 13, HSC's chief of surgery, Blanchard, told Odim he planned to stop the program for six months while assessing the Toronto doctors' report. Blanchard told the young surgeon "he would probably be restarting the program after six months, but without me at the helm," Odim later testified. He also suggested that Odim submit a letter of resignation by the next day. Odim told Blanchard that he had given him too little notice and he said he thought the request for a resignation was "callous and insensitive." He told Blanchard he would not write the letter.

For his part, Odim felt that the mortality rate in 1994 was no different than any of his predecessors. He denied that his surgical skills were at issue. "I would have liked to have seen a lower mortality rate in 1994," he testified. "We all [would have]. When I look at 1993 through 1994 and what the mortality rates are for Winnipeg, the institution, I do not see an appreciable difference. In 1995, twenty per cent of babies under a year who were sent out of province died." The real issue, Odim told the inquest, was the lack of support from his medical team and hospital administrators, which contributed to the high mortality rate of children undergoing heart surgery. Odim eventually resigned in the summer of 1996 and is now working in the United States. As for the inquest, Sinclair won't make his findings known until some time in 1999.

It appears there was a cascade of problems at HSC. First, a pediatric cardiac program was allowed to reopen when there were already worries there might not be enough patients to maintain the skills of the operating room team. Then, a relatively junior surgeon was hired to take over the program, even though he was not rigorously assessed, and lacked a mentor to provide him with a critique of his technical skills. Despite concerns from nurses, anesthetists, and neonatologists, hospital officials did not stop the program or provide it with appropriate support. While these problems were occurring, parents of patients were left with the impression that everything was well and that the surgery was the best the health care system could provide.

Although patients and parents can't possibly be informed of everything, there are many things they should have been made aware of in this case. They should have known not only the death and complication rates of the operations, but the death and complication rates of the *pair of hands* performing the surgery. They should have been made aware of Odim's surgical experience, the number of operations he had performed unassisted, and at least been told that there had been problems with the program in the past. Many would suggest, and appropriately so, that it shouldn't be up to patients or their parents to investigate the surgeon, operating team, and pediatric cardiac program—the system should look after many of those issues. If parents of patients have been made aware of some of the problems, they could have taken their babies elsewhere.

This harrowing story of what occurred in Operating Room 2 at HSC is a horrendous tragedy for these babies and their parents, but it has broader lessons for all hospitals and those who use them. In the most basic terms, no one seemed to be in charge, a situation not unique to Winnipeg. It exists in many hospitals with virtually all surgical and medical procedures. Currently, if members of an operating team suspect there is a quality problem, there is no place to complain and be assured of a thorough, unbiased investigation. Moreover, one might wonder why it should be left to nurses and other doctors in the operating room to complain in the first place. Certainly, there should be a monitoring program that quickly picks up problems as severe as excessive death rates, to say nothing of high complication rates. Learning of these problems in an inquest, while useful, is far too late for some.

## QUESTIONS TO ASK A SURGEON

*As part of informed consent, a physician must explain the procedure to you, informing you of all risks, benefits, and alternatives to surgery. Before consenting to an operation, you should ask:*

- How experienced are you at this surgery?
- How many of these operations have you performed unassisted?
- What are the death and complication rates of this procedure for the hospital? For you individually?
- How do those rates compare to other hospitals?
- Are there other more experienced surgeons who perform this procedure in this hospital?
- Does this hospital have a monitoring system for the performance of the operating room team? If so, what is it and can I see the results?
- What is the hospital process for keeping me informed during the surgery and after?

## THINGS YOU CAN DO TO HELP

- Lobby your federal and provincial governments to ensure that "high-risk" surgeries are done only in hospitals where surgeons and others are able to maintain their skills by performing a lot of them.
- Advocate for a hospital watchdog body that routinely monitors surgery programs and allows nurses and medical staff to voice their concerns and be heard.

*Two*

# Rating Hospitals

Just as consumer guides direct shoppers to the best hotels and restaurants, there are guides to the best doctors and hospitals—in the United States. *Best Doctors in America, America's Best Hospitals, The Consumer Guide to Coronary Artery Bypass Graft Surgery,* and *16,638 Questionable Doctors* are just a few of the books available to savvy health care consumers searching for top-rated hospitals and doctors. Whether these books are put out by government-funded agencies or book publishers, they tell patients how many people have died under a surgeon's scalpel, what the complication rates are, and in some cases, which health care institution has the highest Caesarean section rate. It's a shopper's paradise for patients as they take steps to ensure their bodies are in the safest and most competent hands possible.

In *America's Best Hospitals,* more than 1000 health care

institutions are ranked in areas from "AIDS to urology." *Best Doctors in America* publishes a national compendium of top specialists, based on a reputational survey of physicians. The reputational survey is not scientific but asks top doctors in various specialties this one key question: "If you had a close friend or loved one who needed a neurosurgeon [for example], and you couldn't perform the operation yourself, for whatever reasons, to whom would you refer them?" Those surveyed were promised all comments would remain confidential.

As well, for a fee between $50 to $500 U.S., the Aiken, South Carolina-based company will locate the best specialists for patients' condition, usually those that are "catastrophic" or very serious, such as brain tumours, heart disease, cancer, and AIDS. The pioneer of the company is Greg Smith, who at thirty-four was told he had an inoperable brain tumour and had three months to live. Eleven years later, the Pulitzer prize-winning Smith is alive after locating experts to provide him with experimental therapy. As living proof that patients don't have to accept a death sentence, Smith set up the company to steer others like him to the best specialists. The service is relatively straightforward. "It's bad enough you're been diagnosed with a serious illness. What we do is the work for people, finding the right specialist. All our physicians are on one network," said Christopher Greame, chief operating officer of *Best Doctors*.

One of the first comprehensive guides published, which continues to this day, is *The Consumer Guide to Coronary*

*Artery Bypass Graft Surgery.* Not only is it given out free by the Pennsylvania Health Cost Containment Council, an independent state agency, but its staff once wore T-shirts advertising it under the banner: "Check us out before you check in." And patients have been "checking out" the success rates of 177 cardiac surgeons before "checking into" one of the forty-one state hospitals certified to have doctors perform the surgery for years. Canada has nothing that comes even close to it, even though Ontario, for instance, has the data available to create such a guide.

Patients and others can learn how many operations each surgeon performed, how many died under her or his care, and whether that is considered to be too many. Until the *Consumer Guide* existed, "you didn't know who was excellent, borderline, and who was questionable," said Dr. Ernest Sessa, executive director of the Pennsylvania Health Cost Containment Council. "The good news is that there's some place to look now."

Although many American surgeons initially opposed the publishing of such consumer guides, the results are compelling: since the guide has been made public, death rates for cardiac bypass operations in Pennsylvania have declined by more than one quarter. Specifically, the risk-adjusted mortality rate in Pennsylvania declined from 3.89 per cent in 1990 to 2.85 per cent in 1993. Every year, about twenty-three thousand cardiac bypass surgeries are performed. While a one per cent drop may not sound dramatic, consider this: that decrease means 240 more Pennsylvanians are potentially alive each year from heart operations who previously wouldn't have been. That's the equivalent to a full load of airplane passengers.

New York has had similarly impressive results after being the first in the United States to implement a program of publishing death rates by surgeon, but the difference between its guide and Pennsylvania's is that the latter state publishes every surgeon's name—not just those who performed more than two hundred operations annually. Still, New York has seen dramatic improvements since publicizing the death rates in its own consumer guide: it reported a forty-one per cent decrease in the risk-adjusted mortality rate for cardiac surgery, dropping from 4.17 per cent to 2.45 per cent between 1989 and 1992. That decrease translates into 309 more patients a year who are surviving their surgery. A 1997 *Journal of the American Medical Association* study says that over a five-year period, there has been a fifty-two per cent drop in the cardiac surgery death rate.

Studies have shown that gentle persuasion and the mere publishing of clinical guidelines—a medical recipe of sorts that instructs doctors how to treat patients with a given ailment—doesn't get physicians to significantly change their behaviour. What has proven to work is competition and peer pressure. Publishing not only clinical guidelines but how real patients actually fare after surgery works its own magic in the form of what those in the field call the "shame factor." When risk-adjusted death and complication rates are published by individual physician name, no one likes being at the bottom of the list, particularly not competitive doctors or hospitals in search of patients. "It doesn't work if you try to do it voluntarily [with doctors]. It has to be made public," said Sessa, adding that "you have to give people a reason to change. And the reasons are public accountability and competition."

Information on heart surgeons in New York might never have been published had the newspaper *Long Island Newsday* not gone to court after then senior medical reporter David Zinman was refused the information under the state's Freedom of Information Laws (FOIL). Zinman knew the information existed after hearing that Dr. Mark Chassin, then commissioner of the New York State Department of Health, was telling hospitals they should have more information on individual surgeons. "We found there was enormous variability even after you adjusted for risk factors. You could figure out who was going to die," said Chassin in an interview at Mount Sinai Medical Center in Manhattan, where he currently chairs the health policy department.

Initially, Chassin wasn't keen to have reporters point out to the public which hospital they were most likely to die in. He was worried about the political fallout and suspected the benefit wouldn't outweigh the harm. The state health department also felt officials could remedy the problem through the Cardiac Advisory committee, made up of cardiac surgeons, cardiologists, and general physicians.

Arguing before New York State Supreme Court Justice Harold J. Hughes on why the figures should not be publicly released, the state health department said the data would be of "little public benefit" and would be misused and misunderstood—to the detriment of the physicians identified.

In a strongly worded judgment written on October 15, 1991, Hughes took issue with the state's paternalistic reasoning:

> In other words, the State must protect its citizens from their intellectual shortcomings by keeping from them information beyond their ability to comprehend. Following the department's position to its logical end, it appears that if members of the public were more intelligent, it would be in the public interest to disclose this information. The duty of administrators to release to the population the records of its government cannot be dependent upon the administrators' assessment of the population's intelligence.

Hughes was willing to entertain the notion that releasing the data could be an issue of privacy.

> Here, assuming for the sake of argument that the actions of a physician in his professional capacity are personal ... the issue becomes whether a surgeon operating in a hospital has a legitimate expectation that the results of his surgery will be withheld from the public. He or she does not. A surgeon's work is often monitored by video recording, and is subject to constant peer review. Government agencies ... are always looking over the surgeon's shoulder. Insurance companies have a continuing interest in surgical outcomes. No doctor subject to such scrutiny could have any reasonable expectation that

> the government would withhold from its citizens the patient mortality rate of the doctor. Furthermore, even if there was a legitimate privacy expectation, the interest of the public outweighs it. The Department of Health recognized such by releasing the information to the hospitals so that patients, as consumers, could make a more intelligent decision about which cardiac surgeon to choose. The same public interest compels that the information be made available to the rest of the state.

News of the judgment was greeted with indignation: Some heart surgeons vowed they wouldn't take more complex cases for fear of driving their mortality rates up, while others claimed the health researchers' data were faulty. Rumours of half-dead, elderly patients fleeing to the Cleveland Clinic for surgery as a last resort were rampant, and surgeons complained vigorously that the death rate "adjustments" to account for thirteen different complications in minute detail were inaccurate. Most of those doctors with high death rates—some as high as twenty-one per cent or more than five times the state average—felt it was because they had more complex cases. "There was a lot of scaremongering going on," said Chassin, who studied these allegations to find out their impact on reporting the death rates.

Dr. Sidney Wolfe of Ralph Nader's Public Citizens Health Research Policy in Washington, D.C., criticized surgeons who blasted the system. "It shows they fail to believe or understand the whole process of risk adjustment … . There is no advantage to taking low risk patients, because their condition is taken into consideration when a doctor's mortality rate is risk adjusted … . It is also unethical for physicians to say they won't care for sick patients because they are worried about their mortality rates," he told Zinman.

Thomas Hartman, then deputy director of health care standards for the state health department, also pointed out there was no escaping the numbers or ratings. No surgeon could hide her or his talent with the scalpel by picking patients that weren't very ill. "A surgeon who thinks he or she can score high on the ranking simply by taking easier patients just does not understand the system. Our whole methodology is designed to adjust for severity of illness and eliminate bias against those who perform surgery on sicker patients," Hartman was quoted as saying. Conversely, a doctor who took only high-risk cases could lose several patients without being severely penalized.

Say, for example, a surgeon operated on one hundred high-risk patients. Based on the difficulty of those cases, experts predict ten should die. If ten actually do die, the surgeon's "risk-adjusted" death rate will be the state average for all surgeons. But if another surgeon had only five patients die, that surgeon would be twice as good as the state average.

Since New York State began publishing heart surgery outcomes by doctor and by hospital, overall risk-adjusted death rates for cardiac bypass surgery have plummeted by forty-one per cent. And Winthrop-University Hospital, in

Mineola, Long Island, took its ranking of twenty-ninth out of thirty hospitals in New York State seriously. The only hospital doing a worse job—Erie County—closed down its program. (It has recently reopened with excellent results and is currently a highly-rated institution in New York State.) "Patients were less sick here and they were dying," said Dr. William Scott, chair of the Department of Thoracic and Cardiovascular Surgery at Winthrop-University Hospital.

When the state health department was forced to compel all thirty hospitals providing cardiac bypass surgery to report death rates by surgeon, the public learned Winthrop-University Hospital had an overall "risk-adjusted mortality rate" of 9.56 per cent for the year leading up to March 1990. That means even after health researchers "adjusted" for the severity of cardiac patients, about one in ten still died. That was more than double the 4.17 per cent "adjusted death rate" average for New York State's seventeen thousand adults who received cardiac bypass surgeries in 1990. Put another way, the adjusted mortality rates of Winthrop-University Hospital's surgeons ranged from 2.13 per cent to 18.23 per cent. Four of its eight surgeons had done fewer than fifty operations in each of the two years—the largest number of low-volume surgeons at any hospital. "This was the first time anybody at that level started to hold people accountable for their outcomes. For a long time, there was no accountability," said Scott.

Scott was given the job of turning the program around, and part of fixing the problem was getting rid of and changing the case loads of surgeons. "I told some doctors they were okay to do low-risk cases but they needed better statistics if they wanted high-risk patients," Scott said. "There was no doubt we had a problem. Everybody finally had to agree on it."

Fixing this problem wasn't easy and it came at a price: four new surgeons were hired and four of Winthrop's seven cardiac surgeons were persuaded to move on, including one who had his privileges suspended. "One of them [who voluntarily turned in his surgical privileges] has thanked me a hundred times since then. He said he had knots in his stomach every time he went into the operating room," said Scott. "I changed the case loads of doctors—sometimes it was with some sugar, sometimes it was with a stick." Today, Winthrop is one of the highest-rated New York State hospitals for heart surgery. Hospital officials are so proud of its current ratings, they've taken out full-page ads in the *New York Times* boasting that "over three consecutive years Winthrop's Heart Surgery Program has been recognized by the Department of Health as one of the three best in New York State." The ads say that "Winthrop is the only hospital in the state to achieve this outstanding status for three years running."

Although doctors are getting used to their death rates being published, there still is a backlash by some in the medical profession. Repeated time and time again as fact, these myths are spread by cardiac surgeons and others about the deleterious effects of what are commonly called "surgical scorecards."

- **Myth:** Surgeons in New York are turning away severely ill cardiac patients in an attempt to keep their surgical death rates low.
  **Fact:** New York state surgeons are treating more critically ill patients than ever and they operate on far more elderly patients on a per capita basis than Canada does.

- **Myth:** Critically ill patients in New York State are flocking to the Cleveland Clinic because they can't find a surgeon to operate on them.
  **Fact:** After researchers took a closer look, they found the number of New Yorkers going outside the state for bypass surgery is going down, as measured in the medicare population.

- **Myth:** Surgeons and their respective hospitals get to top of the list with "low death rates" by operating on younger cardiac patients who don't have a lot of complications.
  **Fact:** The opposite is true. Dr. William Scott of Winthrop-University Hospital has an "expected death rate" of 3.34 per cent because his cases are some of the most complex in the state. But his risk-adjusted death rate was one of the lowest in the state at 0.97 per cent. Very often, hospitals who have the lowest risk-adjusted death rates published have the riskiest, sickest patients.

- **Myth:** Publishing names of surgeons and hospitals is useless, as patients don't use the information.
  **Fact:** Although studies have shown that patients primarily rely on friends and family to find a cardiac surgeon,

researchers believe that publishing names of doctors and hospitals appears to have a sentinel or peer pressure effect, thus encouraging officials to "fix" whatever potential problems there are.

- **Myth:** The "risk adjustments" made to correct for doctors who take high-risk patients aren't accurate or fair. **Fact:** New York has thirteen different risk factors to help determine the "risk-adjusted" rates. Pennsylvania has seven, including risk factors such as those patients who have had previous heart attacks, patients with renal failure, those in cardiogenic shock, and women who don't do as well as men after cardiac surgery.

- **Myth:** Patients are being steered by insurance companies to hospitals with the lowest heart surgery prices. **Fact:** High cost does not necessarily mean better quality. Studies have found that hospitals with the worst rates have not lost patients, and oddly, hospitals with the best survival rates have not gained "market share." The Hospital of the University of Pennsylvania, which had more deaths than expected, charged $86,509 for surgery. Lancaster General Hospital charges one-third of the cost, or $29,481, while staying within its "expected death rate." [1993 data]

Chassin ascribes the decrease in death rates—some of which were unusually high in some centres—to improved quality programs and the firing, retirements, and migration of low-volume surgeons, particularly those doing fewer than fifty operations a year. One health researcher who tracked the number of low-volume heart surgeons in New York found that the state-wide death rate dropped significantly when those surgeons moved to other states or retired.

Perhaps one of the most striking features of the reporting program is the way it ferrets out problems in the quality of care that would have never been detected otherwise. This isn't to say that hospitals don't want to unearth these problems, but sometimes those working in hospitals can be so close to a situation that they don't always detect their shortcomings no matter how hard they try.

At one point, St. Peter's Hospital in Albany, N.Y., a 447-bed community teaching hospital, had the third-highest actual death rate in 1991 from cardiac surgery in the state, at 4.6 per cent. However, their "expected death rate" was less than half at 2.1 per cent, suggesting they had a high death rate with low-risk cases. That means that once their cardiac cases were adjusted for risk, one out of fifty patients was "expected" to die from the surgery, but in practice, about one in twenty-two died. "The staff reacted to these figures with frustration and scepticism. There was general agreement that the published results posed a real and serious problem, but some questioned whether the problem was not in the surgery but in the statistics that were thought to underestimate patient risk levels," according to a paper presented by Dr. Stanley W. Dziuban.

A review by a St. Peter's Hospital subcommittee that included chiefs of medicine and cardiology confirmed the opinions of their cardiac surgeons that "there were no identifiable errors in care or any noticeable patterns except that the patients who died were 'very sick and high risk.'" But after closer scrutiny, and with some help from state officials, St. Peter's found that its pre-operative use of the intra-aortic balloon pump, a device that helps the heart circulate blood, was used on less than one-quarter of very sick patients receiving emergency surgery in 1991 and 1992. By the end of 1993, eighty-nine per cent of these patients received the pump, cutting the hospital's death rate in half.

"Do they look at the figures and change?" asked Chassin. "Some do, some don't and that's our challenge. The initial reaction [by doctors] to this sort of information to publish telephone book-sized reports is that it's 'bad science.'" Dr. James Mazzara, chair of the committee on cardiovascular disease at the Medical Society for the State of New York, said publicizing results did nothing to help reduce the death rates. "That information was known even before it was published in a newspaper," said Mazzara, who believes it was the initiatives of hospital staff that helped reduce the death rates. "There's a flurry in the paper for one or two days and then it really has no impact."

Mazzara believes the problems would have been solved by physicians eventually—something Chassin disagrees with. "It's the peer pressure that I think is the engine for people to pay attention to the data," said Chassin. As Arthur Levin, director of the Center for Medical Consumers in New York City, pointed out, "we know providers will kick and scream when this information is released, but it's good public policy ... It's also a question of informed consent. Patients can't give informed consent if they don't know what the risks are."

One would think these guides would be prime reading material for cardiologists, specialists who refer patients to cardiac surgeons. But a study showed that few cardiologists use the scorecards when deciding where to send patients. The study, published in the *New England Journal of Medicine* in 1997, found a staggering "eighty-seven per cent of the cardiologists reported that the [Pennsylvania] guide had a minimal influence or none on their referral recommendations. The majority of the respondents never discussed the consumer guide with their patients undergoing CABG [cardiac artery bypass graft surgery]," wrote Drs. Eric Schneider and Arnold Epstein. In fact, "only two per cent of the cardiologists responded that the consumer guide had a 'significant impact' on their referrals," said the authors, who concluded that the guide has "limited credibility among cardiovascular specialists."

Sessa believes "it's very arrogant [for cardiologists] to ignore a guide like ours." After all, some patients find out they need cardiac surgery only after a heart attack, hardly the time one feels like thumbing through a guide of death rates by surgeon. But that's exactly the time a patient needs a good referral from their cardiologist.

Perhaps it is for this reason alone that the state has had to be a tough-minded advocate for the patient. Hospitals don't have a choice—they have to give out the figures. "If the CEO refuses to give us the data or intentionally gives us wrong data, he could find himself in jail," said Sessa, adding that there is also a $1000-a-day fine for those who fail to comply. As a result, "ninety-eight to ninety-nine per cent of them comply," said Joe Martin, press secretary for the Pennsylvania Health Care Cost Containment Council.

Overall results of New York's and Pennsylvania's publications are enough to suggest that death rates by hospital and by surgeon should be released. They would not only inform the public and unearth quality problems, but would force a higher degree of excellence in cardiac surgery. A similar program could easily be started in Ontario, which collects data in almost the identical way as the United States does. However, although overall figures on cardiac surgery are reported by Ontario's Provincial Adult Cardiac Care Network, it refuses to give out death rates by hospital or by doctor.

The Cardiac Care Network's chair, Barry Monaghan, said it's not necessary to publish complication and death rates for Ontario surgeons because they do many operations and are very proficient at them. However, one might argue, if the figures are as good as experts says they are, then why not release them? It sounds like something Canadians would want to brag about.

"I honestly don't think, in the cardiac area, there is a value added to publishing surgeon-specific rates," Monaghan said in an interview. "We know what the performance of individual surgeons is and if there is an outlier [a surgeon with a higher death or complication rate than the rest], it is shared with the chief" of cardiac surgery at the hospital and any problems are quickly dealt with.

That said, a recent study found that eight heart surgeons in Ontario were performing fewer than one hundred cardiac bypass graft surgeries a year, which is considered by some experts to be low-volume. That includes two surgeons who are doing fewer than fifty of the bypass surgeries a year. The study by Dr. Jack Tu does not say whether these doctors are simply low-volume surgeons or whether they are supplementing their bypass operations with more complex heart-valve replacement surgeries, thus keeping their skills up. Why doesn't the public know that? Wouldn't a patient rather be operated on by the surgeon performing three hundred of these operations a year instead of thirty?

Another thing: According to Freedom of Information and Protection of Privacy Act (FOI) documents, over a fifteen-month period between July 1995 and October 1996, Ontario's cardiac care network had to postpone more than 1000 operations, suggesting that all may not be well for those on heart surgery waiting lists. The most common reasons given for cancelling the surgeries were to operate on more urgent cases, lack of intensive care unit beds, or having no blood products available. "Our cancellation rates have been terrible," said Dr. Bernard Goldman, head of cardiovascular surgery at Sunnybrook Health Science Centre. "What we see are people being admitted to other hospitals with reactive episodes or complaints of heart attacks and unstable episodes of angina." According to

Goldman, "It forces us into a more urgent scenario. It's a nightmare."

Although Monaghan says giving out the numbers of deaths by surgeon isn't necessary, he is coming around to the idea that perhaps the Provincial Adult Cardiac Care Network should consider publishing more data for the public in the form of a report card, especially since Ontario's hospitals are doing such a good job. This may or may not be a difficult task, depending on how averse heart surgeons are to having risk-adjusted death rates published.

Currently, there are no consumer guides in Canada telling patients where to shop for health care, so they are left to ask for advice from friends, relatives, and their family doctors. Although a few Canadian hospitals are named in *America's Best Hospitals,* which is largely based on reputation, there is no comprehensive way for patients to find their way through the maze of complication rates, death rates, how well hospitals discharge patients, or how much nursing care is available. But it looks like that may soon change.

Frustrated by the lack of information available to prospective patients, I conducted a survey of Ontario hospitals as part of of my Atkinson Fellowship in Public Policy. The thirty-eight-question survey was mailed to all Greater Toronto Area acute-care hospitals and others randomly selected in Ontario's six regions for a total of seventy-two hospitals. The survey followed a pilot test of six Ontario hospitals and involved the help of more than twenty people including epidemiologists, surgeons, hospital CEOs, a credentialling lawyer, nurses, administrators, and Toronto

Hospital's chief of surgery Dr. Paul Walker. In all, fifty-three hospitals responded, for a seventy-four per cent response rate—a rate high enough to make generalizations about acute-care hospitals in the province. Nineteen hospital presidents chose not to answer the survey, which included questions on patient satisfaction, how they monitor continuing medical education of physicians, and the complication rates of keyhole bladder operations, to name just a few.

The survey looked at how thoroughly hospitals research doctors before they are extended operating or admitting privileges, whether they insist on having their doctors take continuing medical education courses, how they monitor surgeries and potential complications, whether they track patient satisfaction, and whether the institution is accredited. The survey was not about the safest or most dangerous, or best or worst hospitals. Instead, it focused on how these institutions monitor their services, surgeries, and doctors.

The main findings were that although the vast majority of hospitals ask doctors applying for surgical or admitting privileges whether they have been found negligent in a malpractice suit, three hospitals said they don't. When a hospital grants surgical and admitting privileges, it means the surgeons and physicians are allowed to operate and check patients into a particular hospital. Without these privileges, it is extremely difficult for a physician to practise medicine. Most hospitals want to know if a doctor has been found guilty of injuring a patient or practising bad medicine. Only one hospital didn't ask prospective doctors looking for privileges whether they had been suspended from other hospitals for reasons other than budgetary problems. Eleven hospitals did not monitor if doctors met continuing medical education requirements. Only a few hospitals that monitor continuing medical education take a hard line if doctors do not meet those requirements.

Since hospitals use various methods to measure how satisfied their patients are, it is almost impossible to compare one hospital to the next. However, some downtown Toronto teaching hospitals are trying to change that by having their patients fill out a standard survey. Also, fourteen or one-quarter of hospitals surveyed did not have a designated staff member to deal with complaints, but at those that did, patients overwhelmingly identified communication with their doctor or nurse as the biggest problem. Words such as "rude" or "uncaring" popped up, while others complained about the food, the cost to park, and the length of time they had to wait to see a physician.

When the new surgical technique of laparoscopic cholecystectomy, known as keyhole gallbladder surgery, was introduced to surgeons in the early 1990s, training ranged from hospitals allowing doctors to work on pigs at a weekend course to the endorsement of a very rigorous monitoring process of doctors learning this new surgery that boasted a smaller scar and a shorter hospital stay.

Finally, a surgery to help prevent strokes called carotid endarterectomy was looked at, largely because it is controversial and experts have suggested patients have the best results when the operation is performed by a surgeon who does at least twelve of these operations a year. The operation, performed with varying results by vascular surgeons in Canada and neurosurgeons in the U.S., involves cleaning the plaque out of one or both carotid arteries in the neck (but not at the same time). Despite the worry about low-volume surgeries, the survey found that eighteen out of forty-seven surgeons do less than ten of the procedures in one year. This number includes nine surgeons who performed five or less surgeries a year.

After the Ontario hospital survey was published as part of the Atkinson Fellowship in fall 1997, some hospitals polished up press releases to say they had been recognized as being good institutions, while others discounted the work as unscientific. However, it appeared to garner interest at the Ontario Hospital Association (OHA), which announced shortly after the survey came out that it would be doing its own report cards on hospitals. It is expected to issue its first "report card" on the hospital system in general in the fall of 1998 before moving to reports on individual hospitals some time in 1999 in a undertaking that is expected to cost more than $1 million. At a meeting the OHA voted to "undertake to develop appropriate comparative indicators which will allow residents in Ontario's communities to make informed choices with respect to the outcomes and level of quality being provided by hospitals in Ontario." If all goes well, patients in Ontario will be the first in Canada to be able to shop for a hospital. But the changes don't end there.

The downtown Toronto teaching hospitals are forming

their own report card; a grant has been given to explore the creation of a national scorecard; the Atkinson Charitable Foundation also extended a grant to explore the creation of consumer guides to hospitals, doctors, and community health services; and *Maclean's* magazine has published an issue comparing provinces' health care performance. In addition, the federal government has talked about the need to do report cards on the health care system.

If prospective patients need to know the "bests" in Canadian hospitals in 1998, there is no guide available to them. Instead, they have to rely on word of mouth from friends and relatives, or a strong referral from a family doctor. Our neighbours to the south may not have the best health care system in the world, but they certainly have found the best ways to measure their system and get that information out to consumers, and for this they are decades ahead of Canada. Some have argued these guides only exist because the health care system in the U.S. is competitive and based on a free market, but it would be naive to believe that a strong consumer movement and legislators who feel a moral responsibility to give information to patients were not also key contributing factors.

Sadly, there has not been a strong health consumer movement in Canada equivalent to that of Ralph Nader's group in the United States. As polite Canadians, we haven't demanded more information. Many of us have assumed that since government funds the health care system through billions in tax dollars every year, that funding is equivalent to the Good Housekeeping seal of medical approval. But it isn't, it's merely a promise that the government will act as an insurer, not as quality police.

While many believe the quality of health care to be very good in Canadian hospitals overall, there are too many examples of poor quality of care and patients not being properly informed of risks. Even though there is a lack of publicly available information, there are things you can do to make not only your own stay in hospital better but your health care system better. Ask questions not only of your hospital but of your politicians, and let them know a grass roots health care consumer movement is burgeoning.

## QUESTIONS TO ASK A HOSPITAL

*Millions of Canadians are admitted to hospitals every year but few know just how good those institutions are. Although there are no consumer guides, there are questions you can ask of your local hospital before being treated there.*

- Is this hospital accredited by the Canadian Council of Health Services Accreditation?
- For how many years has it been accredited?
- Does this hospital measure patient satisfaction? If so, can you tell me the results of your recent survey?
- Does this hospital routinely monitor its death and complication rates? If so, how do they compare to other hospitals?
- Have there been any problems between this hospital, the doctor, and the Hospital Appeal Board?
- Has this hospital ever had to suspend this doctor or alter his case load?
- Does this hospital have someone designated to deal with patient complaints? If so, who is it?

## WHAT YOU CAN DO TO HELP

- Lobby provincial and federal governments to make consumer guides for hospitals and doctors the law.
- Push hospitals and governments to have death and complication rates published in a report card.

*Three*

# The "Check-up" for Doctors

Learning details of a doctor's past is a toll-free call away in Massachusetts. By simply dialling a 1-800 number, patients can find out if their doctor has been found negligent in a malpractice suit, settled a case out of court, or garnered a criminal conviction. It's a state-funded service that allows patients to do their own check-ups of physicians and it's in direct contrast to the situation in Canada, where all that information is shrouded in secrecy.

Although this type of consumer service is offered in about a half dozen American states, Massachusetts provides the most comprehensive information to prospective patients under a state law. "There's a public cry for more information on doctors and it's a way of informing people. It's important to know something about the person you're trusting with your most precious possession," said

Kim Hinden, spokesperson for the Massachusetts office of consumer affairs.

The service has been incredibly popular with Massachusetts citizens: since its inception in November 1996, the state had received more than 100,000 telephone inquiries about doctors and more than 1.5 million hits on its Internet site by early 1998. Although the service initially received a fair amount of resistance from the medical profession, doctors are grudgingly in favour of it and even helped the state set it up, despite the constant worry that bad publicity could hurt an individual physician's medical practice.

Although Hinden stresses the service does not provide a complete biography of a given doctor, it does render a medical snapshot. In addition to malpractice findings, settlements, and criminal convictions, the toll-free line also informs patients of any disciplinary convictions by the state medical licensing authority.

Even though patients want the information, not all of them go elsewhere when learning something potentially worrisome about a doctor's past. In one case, a patient found out about a court finding of negligence in a malpractice case through the Massachusetts toll-free line and then went to the doctor and asked him about it. The physician explained what had happened and that the incident had occurred long ago, which was good enough for the patient. The patient made an informed choice after using a consumer protection service that is foreign to Canadians.

Arguably, one of the most important pieces of information about a physician's past to patients is his or her brush with malpractice. A finding of negligence in a malpractice case in Canada means the judge or jury found the doctor provided below a reasonable standard of care to a patient. It does not mean the doctor is dangerous or incompetent, but it frequently means that more than a simple mistake was made. Certain doctors, such as those who operate on patients' brains, bones, and hearts, and those who deliver babies, are sued far more often than other physicians, mostly because they practise some of the riskiest medicine.

If prospective patients want to research whether a physician was found negligent in a malpractice case, they would have to sift through court records in cities and towns across the country, and even then they would find only cases in which there was a judgment made by a judge or jury. If there was an out-of-court settlement, which happens more and more, the public would most likely never learn of it. The only exception is an out-of-court settlement regarding an infant or a patient who has been left mentally incapacitated, as a judge has to approve it in court. Potentially, a doctor could be found negligent in malpractice cases several times over and patients would be none be the wiser.

If that isn't worrisome enough, consider this: Negligence findings aren't forwarded to the doctors' watchdog bodies, the college of physicians and surgeons in each province. Dr. Stuart Lee, secretary-treasurer of the Canadian Medical Protective Association (CMPA), the physicians' malpractice insurer, says they are lawyer-client privilege. That, even though they are findings made in a court. Many would automatically assume the colleges are made aware of these, particularly since they are the regulatory bodies for physicians and deal with issues of quality and competence. But they are not. So while a court finding about a doctor's negligence can be published, it will not necessarily translate into additional training or a restriction of his or her licence to practise medicine.

One of the main difficulties of malpractice is trying to gauge just how rare or widespread it is. No comprehensive study on patients injured by medical care has ever been done in Canada, but several have been undertaken in the U.S., with the Harvard Medical Practice Study, published in the *New England Journal of Medicine* in 1991, being the most frequently cited one. After poring over more than thirty thousand charts in fifty-one New York State hospitals, Harvard researchers found four per cent of patients hospitalized suffered an injury that prolonged their hospital stay or resulted in measurable disability. Fourteen per cent of those injuries were fatal.

Despite the fear of malpractice in the U.S., the Harvard study—commissioned by then Governor Mario Cuomo of New York—found that nearly ninety-eight per cent of all "adverse events due to negligence in our study did not result in malpractice claims … . Why so few injured patients file claims has not been widely researched. Many may receive adequate health or disability insurance benefits and may not wish to spoil long-standing physician-patient relationships. Others may regard their injuries as minor, consider the small chance of success not worth the cost, or find attorneys repugnant," wrote Dr. Localio and other researchers. "A final possible explanation is that many patients may fail to recognize negligent care." They concluded that hospital injuries are a "hidden epidemic."

Dr. A.E. Miller, who practises medicine in Blackfoot, Idaho, wrote an article that questioned the results of the Harvard Medical Practice Study. It is worth mentioning for no other reason than its title: "Doctors are Being Treated like Cockroaches," published by the *Medical Tribune News Service*. Miller said that if the Harvard study was accurate, physicians would be "the third-leading cause of death in America—right behind heart disease and cancer." Despite severe criticism from some in the medical establishment, the Harvard Medical Practice Study is believed to be the most extensive study ever done on medical malpractice, though it was not the first. Other studies documenting hospital injuries stretch back more than three decades.

In one study, Dr. E. Schimmel wrote an article entitled "The Hazards of Hospitalization in the Annals of Internal Medicine," which found that twenty per cent of patients admitted to a university hospital medical service suffered iatrogenic injuries (medical injuries and death), one-fifth of which were serious or fatal. Other studies have shown that patients were given the wrong doses of medications, or inappropropriate doses of drugs. "Given the complex nature of medical practice and the multitude of interventions that each patient receives, a high error rate is perhaps not surprising," wrote Harvard School of Public Health professor Dr. Lucian Leape in an article.

Hospital errors and injuries are not reported in the

newspapers the way burning plane crashes are, presumably because they could occur in any one of 978 health care institutions across Canada and 5000 different locations in the U.S.

In 1994, Leape wrote an article entitled "Error in Medicine," published in the *Journal of the American Medical Association*, which was largely based on the previous Harvard study. If extrapolated and if "these rates are typical of the United States, then 180,000 people die each year partly as a result of iatrogenic injury, the equivalent of three jumbo-jet crashes every two days," Leape wrote. This is also four times the U.S.'s annual automobile accident death rate of 45,000. Put another way, errors in medicine could account for more deaths than all of the other accidents combined in the U.S., according to the Institute of Medicine.

Leape also pointed to a study of intensive care units that revealed an average of 1.7 errors per day, per patient. Although that number of errors meant hospitals were functioning at a ninety-nine per cent level of proficiency, a one per cent failure rate is "substantially higher than is tolerated in industry, particularly in hazardous fields such as aviation and nuclear power," Leape wrote. As researcher W.E. Deming pointed out, even a 99.9 per cent accuracy rate may not be good enough. "If we had to live with 99.9 per cent, we would have: 2 unsafe plane landings per day at O'Hare, 16,000 pieces of lost mail every hour, [and] 32,000 bank checks deducted from the wrong bank account every hour," he said in a written communication.

Although there is no comprehensive study on the

number of patients injured in Canadian hospitals, Robert Prichard, president of the University of Toronto, believes very few patients injured by medical negligence ever receive compensation. In a report he did, when he was dean of law at the University of Toronto almost a decade ago, entitled "Liability and Compensation in Health Care," he concluded, after scrutinizing figures from Sweden and the United States, that the number who receive compensation for malpractice remains modest and is "certainly less than ten per cent of potential viable claims." According to the book *Legal Liability of Doctors and Hospitals in Canada,* "this has led some commentators to suggest that the real medical malpractice crisis is not that there are too many claims, but quite the opposite—there are not enough successful ones."

This goes against the conventional wisdom that doctors are being crushed in Canadian courts and that there is an explosion of flimsy lawsuits south of the border. The CMPA reports that in 1996 it received 5758 patient-related enquiries from its doctors and, in that same year, the number of legal actions commenced against doctors rose to 1415. However, doctors have an impressive batting average in the courts. In 1996, Canadian doctors won 72 out of 101 cases that went to court and 811 cases against physicians were dropped, says Lee. Even though the doctors' insurer is settling more cases—in 1996 it settled 448, up from 334 in 1995 and 290 in 1994—it has a reputation for fighting until the bitter end, and some say these settlements come well down the litigation road.

In 1996, CMPA paid out $101.6 million in court awards and settlements to patients. Also, it spent an additional $60.9 million in legal bills representing doctors in malpractice claims, physicians' college hearings, and hospital matters in 1996. "If we would spend the money we're wasting on litigation on helping victims, everyone except the lawyers would be better off," said Prichard, after being told about these recent figures.

The truth of the matter is that the vast majority of medical malpractice victims never even make it to court. Years of litigation, exorbitant legal costs, and doctors' reluctance to testify against each other form a formidable mountain most injured patients can't afford to climb. "Medical negligence suits are notoriously expensive, and many potential plaintiffs do not have the financial resources to embark upon litigation," according to the book *Legal Liability of Doctors and Hospitals in Canada*, written by Ellen Picard, justice of the Court of Appeal of Alberta, and Gerald Robertson, professor of law and medicine at the University of Alberta. "Even the availability of contingency fees is not the plaintiff's panacea it may appear to be. If the claim is not large, few lawyers will be interested in taking it on contingency. The evidence presented to the Prichard review was that medical negligence claims involving damages of less than $100,000 are routinely discouraged by legal counsel."

Certainly, the biggest hurdle facing patients is the billion-dollar Goliath of the CMPA, the doctors' defence fund which is largely subsidized by the public. It boasted more then $1.26 billion in reserves in 1996, most of it courtesy of taxpayers. As part of an agreement between provincial governments and medical associations, the taxpayers pay the bulk of doctors' malpractice insurance. In Ontario in 1998, for example, taxpayers will spend from a low of $1008 to subsidize malpractice insurance for each general practitioner out of a total fee of $2208 to a high of $24,128 out of a total fee of $29,028 for each obstetrician. These payments are the same whether a doctor has been successfully sued a dozen times or never even had a statement of claim for malpractice. Other provinces have their own agreements, but taxpayers pay the bulk of doctors' malpractice fees. The doctors pay the rest.

For all that money, taxpayers don't get any information on which doctors were found negligent, or who settled out of court, making the return on their multimillion dollar investment each year a paltry one. In short, the odds are stacked against patients, who in an unwittingly perverse way are subsidizing their own difficulties by financing most of the doctors' defence fund.

Jean McGregor from Barrie, Ontario, spent thirteen years, underwent three operations, endured two trials and one hearing, and had an estimated $847,000 in legal expenses just to get a modest judgment for a fractured left hip. That, even though she made six formal and informal attempts to settle for a relatively modest amount of money, including a one-time low offer of $57,000 plus costs and Ontario Health Insurance Plan claims. "The only thing that kept me going was my stubborn Scottish pride. I wasn't going to let them beat me down," McGregor said.

The presiding judge at McGregor's last trial in 1996, which found general surgeon Dr. Alfred Martin Crossland negligent in sixteen different ways, described the lengthy litigation as "all-out warfare," so much so that he took the "rare and exceptional" move of awarding full solicitor and client costs. Experts predict the cost of the two trials and the lawyers and disbursements on both sides may amount to as much as $2.5 million. With interest, McGregor's total damages are expected to total about $325,000 of that amount.

Crossland, who is now deceased, not only failed to tell McGregor of her poor surgical results, he completely abandoned her despite desperate phone calls made on her behalf. "The conduct of the defendant in this case was more than just merely negligent. It was reprehensible and caused the plaintiff more harm than had originally been inflicted on her by the defendant's negligence," Justice Donald Taliano wrote. McGregor had two more operations after Crossland put a plate and screws in her left hip, but it was the third operation, a full hip replacement done by Dr. Michael Ford of the Orthopedic and Arthritic Hospital, that provided the most relief.

Despite her improved condition, McGregor is not the same vivacious, on-the-go woman she used to be. Before the accident, she took courses at Georgian College, did home decorating, and reupholstered furniture—talents she had applied while running an antique business from the late 1960s to the early 1980s. She also did all the cooking and housework, managed a substantial garden, and spent a great deal of time with her grandchildren dancing, singing, playing, and teaching Scottish songs. But after a fall on her kitchen rug at the age of fifty-five, she was in extraordinary pain and her grandchildren didn't come around as much, her marriage was in tatters, and in her darkest, loneliest moments she thought about killing herself.

Even though McGregor defiantly says she would have mortgaged her house to get justice, she probably would not have been able to make it to court if her lawyers, Daniel Monteith and Mark Johnston, had not footed most of the bill. Even the judge noted how difficult it is for patients to get justice when he stated, "in the normal course of events such struggles are quite frequently broken off by a litigant who is unable or unwilling to endure. The war is usually won by attrition."

According to Prichard, who wrote a report on malpractice, forcing injured patients to court is a "third-rate way to help these people. We need an affordable, valuable system of compensation to help these victims." He noted that patients injured at work get compensation, as do those in car accidents, yet there is no such insurance for patients injured during the course of medical treatment.

In McGregor's case, a background check on the surgeon would not have helped her, since Crossland had no outstanding discipline convictions and no history of malpractice judgments. Still, many patients should have that information as they cannot protect themselves any other way. And judging from McGregor's example, they would not be able to afford to fight in court for compensation for injuries.

It is also difficult for the public to learn if a doctor has been convicted of a crime. As we have seen, there is no formal reporting system whereby doctors are required to give the information to the college of physicians and surgeons in each province. The colleges usually learn of a doctor's criminal past in the same way the rest of the public does—through the news media. However, if the disciplinary body does learn of it, they can charge a doctor with professional misconduct.

Still, even when the college does decide to take action, it isn't always immediate. Dr. Neil Miles, a Toronto plastic surgeon, was sentenced to one year in jail after pleading guilty to assaulting his wife, Mary Ann Miles, in January 1993. Miles beat his wife's face so badly she had to undergo plastic surgery for bruises, fractures to her skull, and a bone graft during reconstructive surgery.

In August 1994, the College of Physicians and Surgeons of Ontario's disciplinary committee ordered Miles to appear on charges of professional misconduct "in that he has been found guilty of an offence relevant to his suitability to practise." Miles' college certificate stated that "alternatively, Dr. Miles is alleged to be guilty of professional misconduct ... in that he failed to maintain the standard of practice of the profession in that he engaged in conduct or an act relevant to the practice of medicine, that, having regard to all the circumstances, would reasonably be regarded by members as disgraceful, dishonourable, or unprofessional." But three years later, in 1997, the college still hadn't made a decision on Miles as no hearing had been scheduled. In an interview in fall 1997, Miles said he had managed to turn his life around and had become an ordained Anglican preacher. "Everything is under control now," Miles said. Two months later, in November 1997, he took his own life.

Should patients know if a doctor has been found guilty of beating his wife? Is it relevant to their care? Miles, by all accounts, was an excellent plastic surgeon who specialized in operations of the hand. Was it important for his patients to know he had been jailed? Arguably, it might have been more important if Miles was a psychiatrist, a family physician, or was doing any form of counselling. It's a tough call, but patients should be able to access this information and decide for themselves.

However, Miles' professional worries weren't limited to his violent past. He had other difficulties in addition to the criminal conviction. In the 1980s he was in trouble with Humber Memorial Hospital for failing to organize on-call emergency coverage despite repeated requests to do so. That left nurses scrambling for plastic surgeons when emergency patients rolled through the doors.

These problems reached a climax one night in September 1989, when "four major plastic surgery cases were presented at emergency at the hospital" and "Dr. Miles was found to be on vacation. No plastic surgery coverage had been arranged," according to files. The nursing supervisor in emergency that night had a "disastrous time" getting the four patients into other hospitals that "themselves were put out and tired of having to be the ultimate alternative emergency department for the hospital."

Although there was no dispute over Miles' abilities, Humber Memorial's medical advisory committee felt that there were "unacceptable call waiting times in emergency for plastic surgery patients" and revoked Miles' hospital privileges, which meant he could not practise medicine or surgery in that hospital. Miles appealed the decision to the Ontario Hospital Appeal Board, and in July 1991 it struck down the Humber Memorial decision, saying the hospital failed "in its duties of natural justice and fairness in the matter" by failing to give notice of a hearing to revoke Miles' privileges. Miles was promptly reinstated and the on-call emergency schedule was worked out.

When a doctor's privileges are revoked or suspended, patients rarely learn of it. It's not something that always shows up in a "certificate of standing" from the college of physicians and surgeons, because the regulatory body depends on the physician in question to provide this information. Although revocation of privileges usually means a given physician can't practise medicine in that particular hospital, it doesn't necessarily mean the doctor is barred from practising in another hospital. In one case, an internist suspended from one hospital continues to work in two others in a battle that has been raging for almost a decade. The doctor's privileges were revoked in 1989 after a hospital's board of governors made a finding of general incompetence. That move followed a report that stated there were more than fifty incidents on which to base the conclusion that the doctor in question "showed an inability to recognize the severity of patients' illness and to institute appropriate care in an appropriate time frame, and that this has sped up or has been the cause of the demise of patients." The shortcomings at the hospital included a "litany of poor charting, poor choice of antibiotics and medication, with critically ill patients."

There were also complaints that the internist "missed or failed to note the fact that the patient had eight broken ribs," and that he failed to notice neck rigidity in a fifteen-year-old later diagnosed with meningitis. A tribunal set aside revocation and ordered a suspension instead, but little has been resolved. Furthermore, an assessment by the College found the internist to be competent. The doctor in question says that hospital officials essentially went on a "rampage ... . There have been false statements made about me. It is totally unfair the way it's being handled." The case continues.

But the only way patients would learn this information is by doing a thorough search of Hospital Appeal Board documents, and they would only find it because the physician challenged the hospital's case.

"It certainly is hard to get rid of doctors," said lawyer Rino Stradiotto, who has represented hospitals trying to do just that. "I tell them [hospital officials] right off the bat, it's going to be contentious, very expensive, and time-consuming. They can count on about two years and $200,000. We've come to a point in society where we favour the individual's rights over the public's rights." Or, in the case of hospitals, individual physicians' rights are favoured over those of patients.

Part of the reason it is so difficult to change the case loads or revoke the privileges of physicians found to fall below an acceptable standard is the Public Hospitals Act. There was a time when a doctor who didn't belong to the right country club, or who was Jewish, or who didn't have great connections had a difficult or impossible time getting privileges at a hospital. The Public Hospitals Act was designed more than two decades ago in Ontario to stifle the old boys' network and make it fairer for doctors to obtain and keep their privileges. However, the act is now being used so that doctors can hold up the process of having their case loads changed or their privileges suspended or revoked literally for years, while patients are none the wiser. Similar legislation exists in other provinces.

That's in contrast to the American courts, which have clearly stated that hospitals owe a duty to their patients to ensure that the physicians to whom privileges are granted are competent. Further, hospitals have a continuing duty to ensure those physicians remain competent through the period during which the privileges apply. In Canada, lawyer Eric Hoaken said, "There is no authority dealing with the specific nature of the duties ... owed by a hospital to a patient directly."

And it's important for hospitals to judge a doctor's medical abilities, as patients can't always know the difference between good and bad hospital care. Elinor Caplan, Health Minister in Ontario in the 1980s, was made aware of one doctor who "always cut through the urethra during a D&C [dilation and curettage, a routine gynelogical procedure].

He was a fellow with a shaky hand. In the lounge, they [other physicians] would joke about who was doing the repairs." But it wasn't a joke for the women who were made incontinent by his quivering knife. (During a D&C, a curette is inserted into the uterus to scrape away the lining.)

The congenial surgeon told these women there was a nick to the urethra and this was a normal complication. The women accepted it, not knowing otherwise. "He had a wonderful bedside manner. And women often referred their friends to him," said Caplan, who is currently a Member of Parliament. The real problem was that these patients "didn't have the ability to make a proper judgement. This doctor had hacked them to bits, but he had a good bedside manner." The doctor was eventually removed from the hospital, despite protests from female patients who thought he was wonderful.

As Hilary Short, the Ontario Hospital Association's vice-president of public affairs and education, points out, "Once you've granted a physician privileges, he has to be falling down drunk every day before you can get rid of him." It's an especially difficult problem for smaller, rural hospitals that may not be keen to challenge the doctor, as they are afraid no one better will want to take his or her job.

Instead of revoking a doctor's privileges and being guaranteed a long fight, hospitals are now being encouraged to pull substandard physicians aside and give them a "heart to heart" talk, which not only helps the physician in question save face, but prevents a report to the college for potential disciplinary action. "The physician could say it was malicious to report to the college. You've got to be very careful. Otherwise you could find yourself in a libel or slander action for reporting," Rino Stradiotto told a winter 1997 conference.

One female hospital executive said she felt uncomfortable that a potentially dangerous or incompetent doctor could quietly take his or her skills to another hospital after the "heart to heart" talk. Stradiotto called it a conundrum. The doctor may be quickly accepting blame because he or she has been caught and would rather move on. "There's no question this creates a moral, ethical responsibility. I don't know if there's a clear-cut solution," he said, adding that hospital executives "have a responsibility to each other. This doctor can't go hospital shopping and take his incompetence to another hospital."

Stradiotto, who has acted on behalf of many hospitals, said: "A high mortality rate and high infection rate are not enough to get rid of a physician." If they aren't enough, how are patients able to protect themselves? Once again, the public reporting of these rates could help, but it would not help officials to deal with the problems that dramatically affect the quality of their hospital.

Besides the question of what hospitals do when they learn of a problem with a doctor, there is also the question of how thoroughly they check out physicians before extending surgical or admitting privileges to them. While most hospitals are supposed to do a painstaking check of past complaints, malpractice suits, and criminal convictions, not all do, nor are they compelled to.

One recommendation of a coroner's jury probing the death of a thirteen-day-old boy, Thomas McGregor, was that hospitals do a better job of reporting and checking up on doctors seeking privileges and that they fully inform patients of the level of care and services they provide. That suggestion followed a jury's examination of the 1996 death of Thomas, who suffered massive brain injuries due to a lack of oxygen after his shoulder became stuck in the birth canal, which is medically referred to as shoulder dystocia. He died after being taken off a respirator.

Much of the inquest centred around the hospital's hiring of the McGregor family's obstetrician, Dr. Christine Bloch. The jury had been told that Sydenham District Hospital in Wallaceburg, Ontario, was without an obstetrician for at least four months until it hired Bloch in 1994. Sydenham's credentials committee favoured granting Bloch privileges before obtaining a letter from her former chief of staff, who later recommended against hiring her, and without obtaining a certificate of professional status from the College of Physicians and Surgeons of Ontario. Those two things are thought to be a routine part of the check hospitals do before extending privileges to a doctor.

For her part, Bloch later testified that she did not hide her past from Sydenham District Hospital when she sought privileges there in 1994. The obstetrician provided the hospital with references, proof of her licence to practise, and the names of Oakville-Trafalgar Memorial Hospital's chief of staff and head of the obstetrics department. She did admit to having "difficulty" with some cases during the year she worked at Oakville-Trafalgar Memorial Hospital in 1993. In fact, several formal complaints and two malpractice suits had been filed against her. One baby died; another is brain damaged. Although Bloch acknowledged she was under some pressure to do vaginal and forceps deliveries at the Oakville hospital to bring down its Caesarean section rate, she said: "I do take responsibility for decisions I made taking care of patients." She also said, "Everyone in Wallaceburg knew everything about my past."

At the inquest, Martha McGregor said she had had three miscarriages, then finally became pregnant through *in vitro* fertilization. She purposely chose Bloch because she wanted an obstetrician to deliver her baby, but Bloch left the hospital before McGregor went into active labour. A family doctor delivered the eleven-pound baby boy and ran into trouble when the shoulders became stuck in the birth canal. Thomas ultimately emerged blue and unconscious. It was nearly forty-five minutes before he was able to breathe on his own and by that time, he had already suffered brain damage. The jury ruled in November 1997, that Thomas's death was accidental.

Although Bloch was not present at the birth, her training and judgement were critical issues at the inquest. Martha McGregor was quoted in *The Toronto Star* as saying that she wished she had had more information about the obstetrician: "I still strongly believe that had I had the information about Dr. Bloch's credentialling and her history in Oakville, I would never have been in Wallaceburg."

In winter 1998, shortly after the inquest, the College

of Physicians and Surgeons of Ontario referred charges alleging that Bloch had committed professional misconduct to its Discipline Committee. The charges allege that she failed to maintain the standard of practice and "displayed in her professional care a lack of knowledge, skill or judgement or disregard for the welfare of patients." College spokesperson Jim Maclean said he was not at liberty to say which case, or cases, related to the charges being laid.

The jury is still out on Bloch. Whether there is any merit to criticisms made by patients will ultimately be decided by the College of Physicians and Surgeons of Ontario's Discipline Committee, the doctor's watchdog body. For her part, Bloch was quoted as saying "my qualifications didn't have anything to do with this child's death."

If hospitals thoroughly checked a doctor's past, if they could promptly suspend or revoke the privileges of physicians proven to be providing substandard care, if they and the colleges routinely tracked and acted on findings of negligence in malpractice cases, one could easily make the argument that it wouldn't be necessary for patients to need extensive information on their doctors. But those are a lot of ifs.

Though most hospitals do check a doctor's past, others do not, and patients don't know which group their hospital falls into. Even when hospitals do a thorough check of physicians, they can still encounter huge legal difficulties when trying to change the case loads or to suspend or rid themselves of doctors they have found to not be performing to a basic standard. Hospitals have to use their own funds from their operating budgets to fight the case, while some doctors can rely on the largely government-funded CMPA, which represented physicians in 181 hospital matters in 1996. It also represents doctors who are called before their college disciplinary bodies—2131 hearings in Canada alone in 1996.

Instead of subjecting hospitals to endless litigation when they try to alter or revoke a doctor's privileges, there should be legislation making it mandatory for the issue to be settled within thirty days with the balance of probability tilted towards protecting patients. But improvements could be made well before these cases get to the stage of revoking or suspending a doctor's surgical or admitting privileges. Instead of compelling hospital administrators to prove that a doctor is incompetent, doctors' privileges should automatically lapse after a given time period, say every three years. Doctors eligible for the three-year evaluation would be those who have already completed three successive one-year appointments, where they were reviewed by a department chief or a chief of staff. Department chiefs who have concerns about doctors applying for privileges could place the physicians on a one-year probation period. These measures would ensure a doctor would have to meet certain criteria to get privileges back, just as if he or she was reapplying for a job.

As part of that reapplication process, a hospital could insist that a doctor or surgeon meet certain requirements for the position, including having an acceptable death rate, infection rate and readmission rate subject to the specialty he or she is working in. Those "acceptable" rates would be determined by specialists in the field. Consequently, a physician who had an unacceptably high death rate that could not be explained by a case mix of severely ill patients alone could face retraining or dismissal. So, too, could a doctor whose patients developed unusually high numbers of infections or complications after any medical procedure, or who were given the wrong medications.

For extra measure, doctors would have to meet certain continuing medical education requirements in order to keep their hospital admitting privileges or job. If a doctor did not keep current and fulfil a required number of hours of continuing medical education acceptable to the hospital, that could be the cause for retraining or dismissal. These measures would help ensure that doctors stayed up to date.

Where it gets very complex, though, is in the case of malpractice, since the problems aren't limited to patients' lack of awareness of negligence findings and out-of-court settlements by doctors. In addition, patients who wish to sue encounter huge difficulties and financial obstacles. Some experts have suggested no-fault insurance, while others aren't as specific but point out the need for a compensation system for patients injured during the course of medical treatment.

With so many areas where there are no checks and balances in the hospital and regulatory system, patients once again are left without crucial information. A state-mandated, toll-free telephone line like the one in Massachusetts would be a great public service to health care consumers in Canada. But in the meantime, in this country, it's a case of patient beware.

## RESEARCH TO DO AND QUESTIONS TO ASK

*In Canada, there is no one place where patients can do check-ups on their doctors. But here are some questions to ask and ways to find out more about your physician.*

- Call the College of Physicans and Surgeons in any province and ask if there are any disciplinary convictions on the doctor's record.
- Ask the college what hospital the doctor is registered as having privileges at and request that they mail that information out to you. (In some provinces, the document is called a "certificate of status of registration.")
- Once you have obtained that information, telephone the hospital. Ask if the doctor has privileges there and if they are restricted in any way.
- Also ask the hospital when the doctor's privileges were last reviewed and what criteria the physician had to meet to maintain privileges.
- Legal searches are laborious but possible at the courthouse. Look up the physician's name in the general division/civil actions of the provincial court house for malpractice claims and judgments.
- If you feel comfortable, you could ask the doctor if he or she has ever settled out of court or been found negligent in a malpractice case. (This could be a conversation stopper.)

## THINGS YOU CAN DO TO HELP

- Advocate that a toll-free telephone line be set up to provide information on doctors, be it criminal convictions or findings of medical malpractice.

- Lobby the provincial and federal governments to make findings of negligence in malpractice cases public information reportable to the College of Physicians and Surgeons in your province.
- Ask your government, hospitals, and provincial medical association to develop a fair, effective, and standardized system for doctors to maintain their hospital privileges.
- Demand that governments review the medical malpractice system so it is accessible and fair to patients.

*Four*

# The Waiting Game

Unlike the United States, which rations health care by how much people can afford, Canada rations health care by how long people wait. Thousands of patients are on waiting lists for surgeries and diagnostic procedures in Canada, yet most don't know exactly when they will be called or if the sickest are seen the soonest. That's because there is no formal system that tracks how long people queue. Instead, individual hospitals and doctors keep their own lists. Despite the abundant horror stories about waiting lists, they aren't a bad thing in themselves.

If there was no such thing as waiting lists, hospitals would need to have hundreds if not thousands more beds, more doctors, and other staff—just so they would be on hand *in case someone needed them.* On the face of it, that sounds incredibly convenient for patients. But just think about the down times where there isn't a crush of patients needing care: Lots of empty beds, surgeons twiddling their thumbs waiting for someone to walk in, and a health care system that is totally inefficient, to say nothing of wildly expensive. Doctors wouldn't be able to maintain their skills and they would be faced with the temptation of having to perform more procedures on patients just to keep busy. With finite funding there are finite resources. The real problem is that no one seems to manage most of the waits or even knows how long they are. And that's when it gets really scary. Some people wait longer than it is safe for them to do so, while others suffer the inconvenience of having their surgery or diagnostic tests postponed several times.

It's when patients get their operations postponed, when no one tracks why some patients are waiting longer than others, that waiting lists get their bad rap. Some people die, many are in pain, most are anxiously awaiting word on when their operation or diagnostic procedure will be rescheduled. People associate waiting lists with a bad health care system, when the only thing really wrong with them is that they are so poorly organized the sickest can't always get to the front of the line.

In fact, a study prepared for the federal government in 1998 showed that the same five medical procedures—cardiac care, radiation treatment for cancer, cataract surgery, magnetic resonance imaging, and hip and knee replacements—have the longest waiting lists right across the country. Study author Dr. Sam Shortt, Queen's University health policy research unit director, said these waits could be better managed if the suffering of patients was ranked.

•

Nowhere were the problems of long waits clearer than when I spent a year following Ron Marston of Oshawa, who was on the waiting list at Toronto's Orthopedic and Arthritic Hospital for a double knee replacement. Marston had been placed on the waiting list on September 30, 1996, at age sixty-four. He had been experiencing aches and pains in his knees, a result of his treatment plan for ulcerative colitis, which included thirty-five years of steroid medication. Doctors suspected the medication had had the downside of eroding the cartilage in both of his knees. His surgery was scheduled for April 2, 1997, a date he found acceptable.

A University of Toronto survey published in the *New England Journal of Medicine* found that the majority of Canadians queuing for knee replacement surgery thought their waiting times were acceptable. But it is hard to understand exactly what patients find satisfactory, as some may breeze through the waiting time and use it as a period to prepare themselves psychologically, while others can't work and eventually lose their jobs. Others languish at home, only to have their condition worsen.

By late November 1996, Marston's pain had become more intense and the discomfort had begun to rob him of his sleep. Making it up and down the stairs of his two-storey home was becoming such a chore, Marston had to think twice before doing it.

Around that time, he occasionally went to the Oshawa Seniors Centre, one of the five hundred people a day who went through its doors. There, those aged fifty-five years and older gather to do ceramics, attend exercise classes, take Tai Chi, have lunch, and exchange wallet-sized pictures of their grandchildren. "I think he likes it because of all the women there," his wife, Lois, quipped.

Despite these bursts of enjoyment, Marston's condition was deteriorating, and it felt worse in the deep freeze of Canadian winter. Although he had to give up most of the things he loved, such as gardening and golfing, Marston figured that wasn't too bad since it was winter and certainly by spring he would be up and running. Only three or so months to go, Marston figured, but a telephone call from the hospital in early January informed him that there had been a change: his operation was to be delayed two weeks, unless, of course, he wanted to change surgeons and keep closer to his original surgery date. He opted to wait the extra time, and his surgery was rescheduled to April 16. Although Marston initially said he wasn't that irritated with the postponement of his surgery, shortly after he said: "If it gets cancelled one more time, I'm going to start hollering."

Soon the pain was excruciating, and by the end of January 1997, Marston was counting the days. The pain was now radiating to his hands, and it seemed that every part of his body hurt. By late February, the discouragement began to seep in and Marston felt like he couldn't bear it any longer. "I'm counting down the days now. The legs are really bad. Some mornings, I just don't want to get out of bed. I'm getting discouraged," Marston said. The surgery couldn't come soon enough.

The pre-operative appointment at the Orthopedic and

Arthritic Hospital on March 19, 1997, gave Marston hope that the surgery really was going to happen. After some blood was taken, Marston was sent across the street to see Dr. Joel Maser, who specializes in internal medicine. Maser explained the pre-operative appointment was necessary because "we don't like any surprises."

Before this pre-operative program was established, one out of every six patients had had their surgery postponed due to complications such as high blood pressure. It was at this appointment that Maser learned his new patient wasn't so new to surgery. Marston rambled off his surgically removed organs with the cool recital of a grocery list: His appendix, gall-bladder, large colon, and spleen had all been extracted during a seven-hour operation—double the time and far more organs than he had expected would be removed. Marston explained that he had gone into the hospital for the removal of his colon, damaged from ulcerated colitis, but then "my spleen ruptured at the time. They nicked it or something. What am I supposed to do? Sue?" Marston asked. After that operation, Marston had had another surgery to have his rectum and anus removed. Lois often joked that Marston couldn't have any more operations—as there was nothing left to take out. "What he's got left, he's got to keep," she said.

After undergoing a cardiogram, pulmonary function test, blood pressure check, and a few other tests, Marston was told he was in good shape for surgery. True, he had gained a few pounds—he was up to 208—but that was due to his not being able to exercise. "You'll find six weeks after the operation, you've never been better. Your life will be back on track," Maser told Marston. "You'll be independent—you'll have your life back."

After hearing that news, it was on to see nurse Bruce Weber, located in the hospital's main building. In a tiny office, Weber explained how Marston's new knees would be surgically implanted. "You have no doubt worn out all your cartilage," said Weber, using a plastic set of knees to show Marston where they had worn out. "I think you can expect a good ten or twenty years with your new knees."

Made of titanium, a lustrous metal resistant to corrosion, the replacement knees would be fitted into Marston's sawed-down knees. Titanium is used to alloy aircraft metals for low weight, strength, and high-temperature stability, but Marston wouldn't be flying through his rehabilitation. "Knees take work," Weber explained. "It's your job to get them bending."

Four weeks later, on April 16, 1997, Marston lay outside the operating room in a bed in the hall, waiting to be wheeled in. By the time his operation rolled around, he had been waiting 197 days. The operation went smoothly and quickly: seventy-nine minutes to do the first knee, sixty-three minutes to do the second. (The time on the first knee was longer because Marston was taking part in a study and some fluids had to be removed from his knee area.)

All Marston remembered was waking up in a hospital room with his wife and daughter by his side. Within days, the duo prodded Marston to get out of bed to bend his knees. "The pain is just unreal when you get out of bed," he said. "But I'm doing the exercises." Bending the knees shortly after an operation is important, as it helps prevent scar tissue from getting inside the joint.

A week or so later, Marston was transferred to St. John's Rehabilitation Hospital, a North York hospital set on rambling grounds of lush green grass. After spending three weeks at St. John's, Marston was ready to go home—provided he became an outpatient at his local hospital.

A full year after being placed on the waiting list, Marston was finally ready to go back to his old life of volunteering, seniors' committees, golf, travelling, and spending weekends at his cottage in Haliburton. Although his knees still get sore when he drives for long periods, he walks well without the aid of a cane or crutches. Thinking back, Marston thinks maybe he should have put up a bit more of a fuss. "I think I should have started hollering a lot earlier," said Marston. Although he was very pleased with his surgery and subsequent care, "six months is too long to wait. Patients shouldn't have to wait longer than three."

Marston's travels through the waiting list are typical of many patients, although some wait substantially longer, and a few others undergo surgery in a shorter amount of time. Although waiting lists are necessary in a publicly funded system, there comes a time when the personal and social costs are too great, as patients end up sick in hospital and others are off work or on medication for long periods. For others, their conditions worsen, costing more in the long run. Marston was on pain medication and couldn't do his volunteer work; his life was virtually on hold until he had his knee replacements. It wasn't the type of retirement he had dreamed of.

Dr. David Naylor, then chief executive officer of the Institute for Clinical Evaluative Sciences in Ontario, which tracks the use of health care services in that province, said these patients are being let down at the end of their lives. "We're dealing with elderly citizens who have paid taxes for fifty years. They should have a few years of pain-free existence, rather than spending two years sitting stiff and disabled with nightly pain."

Some patients believe a complaint to the hospital president can help, while others say having a medical "in" can help zip them through the waiting list. Lobbying or having a family member who acts as an advocate can also work a little magic. One Metropolitan Toronto woman recommended that those seeking hip replacement surgery—which has some of the longest waits in the country—"shop around" by calling orthopedic surgeons in search of shorter waiting lists. She did and was able to reduce her eighteen-month wait to three weeks. Her advice: "You have to be willing to use the phone." If orthopedic surgeons published their individual waiting lists, patients could at least look around for a doctor with the shortest wait, but Dr. Henry Hamilton, president of the Ontario Orthopedic Association, doesn't think publishing waiting lists would help much. "It's not as if we're being worked to death in the operating room," said Hamilton. He said more money from government is what would really shorten waiting lists for hip and knee replacements.

Others believe that prospective patients shouldn't have to make inquiries themselves. First, how would a patient get a list of orthopedic surgeons? Second, if it's a general practitioner's job to do the surgical referral, why isn't he or she checking waiting lists for the patient? And third, this all assumes that receptionists answering the phone for these orthopedic surgeons are keen to give out their waiting lists to prospective patients.

One hospital that's trying to change the unfairness of waiting lists is Queen Elizabeth II Health Sciences Centre in Halifax, where doctors and others have done a pilot project with an eye to creating a standardized waiting list for orthopedic patients, particularly those who are getting hip and knee replacements. If successful, it would be the first hospital in the country to have standardized waiting lists, where the sickest are seen the soonest. By standardizing waiting lists, researchers and doctors develop a formula for who gets care and when. The amount of pain and loss of mobility are just a couple of areas they are looking at. "The real issue is that orthopedists need a reliable waiting list assessment tool," said Halifax orthopedist Dr. Michael Gross. And that can only be done if there are specific criteria to grade patients on the amount of disability and sickness they are experiencing.

One other problem standardized waiting lists would solve is unfairness. Without knowing the waiting lists for procedures by hospital and by surgeon, there is no way to track whether some patients are jumping the queue. Naylor says he is deeply concerned about some of the extremely long waiting times that have emerged in Canadian health care: "I see them in absolutely nobody's interest." He believes it would be "healthy for us to have publicity about different waiting times by surgeons for different types of procedures, not only for orthopedic surgeons but for cataract surgery and a host of other procedures where we seem to have long waiting times." If doctors and hospitals published waiting lists by doctor and operation, it would allow patients to shop around, thus naturally cutting down on some of the extraordinarily long waits.

No matter which way you slice it, the figures are startling. Statistics Canada reported in 1991 that forty-five per cent of those who are waiting for health care in this country describe themselves as being "in pain." While not all of their pain would be alleviated by a visit to the doctor or by the surgical procedure for which they are waiting, some of it is presumably due to queuing for care. More than one million Canadians felt they needed care but did not receive it in 1994, including thirty per cent of those in moderate or severe pain, according to the Statistics Canada National Population Health Survey, 1994-95.

A 1996 national survey of the College of Family Physicians of Canada found general practitioners are concerned about the effects queuing for care has on their patients. Almost forty per cent of the one thousand family doctors surveyed said they have to spend at least three hours a week battling bureaucracy while trying to care for their patients. And almost nine in ten family physicians said patients are put at risk or are potentially endangered by having to wait for tests, surgery, and some medical treatments.

The Fraser Institute wrote a report entitled *Waiting Your Turn: Hospital Waiting Lists in Canada,* which estimated that 172,766 people queued for surgical procedures in 1996, up from the Institute's 1995 estimate of 155,969. "Not only were there approximately 11 per cent more people waiting for treatment than there were in 1995, but those waiting were waiting longer to receive their treatment—10.9 weeks from referral to a specialist by a general practitioner to the receipt of treatment, compared to 10 weeks in 1995."

Although the Fraser Institute must be credited with pushing waiting lists into public consciousness, their survey response rate is low—averaging thirty-one per cent. That's still far higher than the five to ten per cent frequently encountered by most who mail out surveys, but it's far below the desirable seventy per cent response rate—a rate strong enough to make generalizations about waiting lists and good enough to get published in medical journals. Still, the Fraser Institute's researchers mail out 8700 questionnaires to doctors across the country each year, something no one else has attempted to do. "We don't say we're getting scientifically accurate responses, we're just trying to give some regional depictions," said Cynthia Ramsay, noting that the Institute "has shown that there's not equal access in Canada."

According to the Institute's 1996 publication, queues had improved, with fewer patients waiting, but still there was "an indicator that rationing is taking place." Fraser

Institute executive director Michael Walker said, "the data clearly show that equal access to medicare in Canada is a myth. The number of people on surgical waiting lists and the amount of time they are waiting for treatment varies substantially from province to province."

Of all the provinces in Canada, Nova Scotia is the only one that actually knows what its waits are. That's because Dr. David Elliott measured the one hundred most common medical procedures performed in Nova Scotia over four years. His 1996 government report, *Reporting Health Performance,* noted that "the issue of patients' rights to all information necessary to make an informed decision regarding treatment raises some important considerations for the health care system, and for physicians in particular."

The report found some increases in Nova Scotia waiting times, including those in ear, nose, and throat and eye surgeries. However, many procedures, including hysterectomies, gall-bladder removal, general surgery, and cardiac surgery saw decreases in waiting times over the four-year period. Overall, Elliott found that "waiting times have remained the same or are slightly better than they were several years ago."

Although there have been many complaints about excessively long waits for hip and knee replacements in Nova Scotia, Elliott found that from 1993 to 1996 the wait for an orthopedic surgeon actually decreased. Waits were still substantial, with patients in the queue for an average of about one hundred days, but doctors were doing more surgeries than ever in that province. In reality, orthopedic surgery had the largest increase in number of performed surgeries compared to any other procedure studied, with more than 4200 surgeries performed in 1995-96. In all, the study tracked 347,000 services for the top one hundred surgical procedures, covering three-quarters of all major surgeries since 1992.

Elliott's survey was not embraced by the medical community, especially not by orthopedists whose own personal experiences contradicted Elliott's data showing that waits for hip and knee replacements were coming down. Long-time Halifax orthopedic surgeon Dr. David Petrie called the report bogus. "I can't work any harder without dropping dead," Petrie was quoted as saying in *The Halifax Daily News*. "This is fallacious, quite frankly." Petrie said his patients wait about nine months for hip and knee operations—about three times longer than the report's figures. Some charged that the tracking time of the waits weren't accurate, as patients were subjected to more than one wait: patients wait to see their general practitioner, then wait weeks or months to see a specialist. It's only at the appointment with the specialist that patients are put on the waiting list for surgery, and the earlier waits are difficult to track.

At the time, Health Minister Bernie Boudreau said the report revealed that there has been a two to three per cent increase in the volume of procedures done annually and that the health care system wasn't nearly as sick as some had suggested. "There is no medical system in this world, not now or ever, that will not have waiting times ... particularly in relation to elective procedures," Boudreau told reporters. So-called elective procedures are those where patients are deemed to be healthy enough to wait for the surgery. According to Boudreau, "We feel that in most areas, we're within acceptable limits. There are some areas that need work ... that send a little signal to us." He called the report a good launching pad for correcting problems, "not based on some anecdote that my next-door neighbour's second cousin's mother had to wait X number of days for a particular procedure, therefore we should plunge all sorts of additional money into this area."

There are some patients, even some physicians, who believe that a short wait means the surgeon probably isn't very competent, instead of thinking that the doctor is establishing his or her practice or isn't an avid self-promoter. Some new orthopedic surgeons have three- to four-week waits compared to their more senior colleagues with two-year waits. As orthopedist Dr. Michael Gross of Halifax pointed out: "There are some orthopedic surgeons who are very good at self-marketing but their competency may be suspect."

Also, in Canada, many assume that a long waiting list is somehow the government's fault; that bureaucrats aren't funding the system enough. But there is a dark side to waiting lists: "Unfortunately, I have also met providers [doctors] who take a sort of perverse delight in having a long waiting list. They see it as a mark of their own status and competence. It also becomes a political club that can be used to beat governments and administrators to get more funds," said Naylor.

Whatever its flaws, Elliott's study shows that a province can track its waiting list by procedure if it chooses to, notwithstanding the complexity, time, and labour required to do it. And if that is possible, why not publish waiting lists by hospital and by surgeon in every province so patients can choose a shorter queuing time if they wish? Worry that doctors with shorter waits could be perceived as less competent is not a good reason to keep the public uninformed. Patients may think a doctor with a shorter waiting list is merely available, not incompetent. And if the medical profession believes such doctors may not be competent, then that is an issue for the disciplinary body or hospital to deal with.

There are other reasons why publishing waiting lists would be difficult. First, a standard and uniform method of maintaining waiting lists would be needed so patients could make comparisons between hospitals. It would take work to get the waiting lists in good enough shape to publish, but that shouldn't be a reason to not do it. The other problem is that once waiting lists are published by hospital and by doctor, the provincial and federal governments would be forced to put more money into fixing the excessively long queues. "Using waiting lists as an indicator of lack of access to health care services is a controversial issue," according to a memo prepared for the federal government's Paul Genest in August 1996 and obtained under the federal Access to Information Act. Written by Assistant Deputy Minister André Juneau of Health Canada's policy and consultation branch, the memo said, "In Canada, a choice has been made to deal with the allocation of finite, publicly funded health care resources with queues. We have chosen to manage delays for health care services rather than to actually deny needed care to some."

Still, there is a need to make waiting lists not only fair but shorter, especially in areas such as hip and knee replacements, cataract removals, and magnetic resonance imaging, particularly when the condition of patients could worsen during the time they are queuing for care. It's simply in no one's interests to have ailing patients waiting months on end, unable to work and in pain.

Some suggestions to fix the long queues for care include:

- Standardized waiting lists would allow patients to be assigned a priority based on their severity of illness and disability and would ensure the sickest are treated the soonest.
- To assist in these standardized waiting lists, a database should track these patients to ensure that no one falls through the cracks. When a surgery is cancelled, for example, a health worker should telephone the patient and let him or her know where he or she is on the list and when the operation is going to be rescheduled, even if that means being switched to another surgeon.
- Doctors, politicians, and members of the public should decide how long is "too long" to wait and what should be done if there are excessively long waiting lists.

Today, when patients are placed on Canada's notorious

"waiting lists" they venture into the great unknown. Since patients pay into medicare with their tax dollars, it's not asking too much to know how long the waits are so they can make smart choices. Publishing waiting lists would also have the added bonus of encouraging hospitals to get their excessively long waits down, as prospective health care consumers could vote with their feet.

## QUESTIONS TO ASK WHILE ON A WAITING LIST

*First, make sure you need to be on one. With surgeries that have particularly long waits, such as hip or knee replacement surgery, you may be able to find a surgeon able to do the operation in a shorter time.*

- How long will the wait be?
- Where exactly am I on the waiting list?
- What are my chances of having my surgery cancelled?
- Will the wait affect my chances of recovery?
- What are my chances of dying while on the waiting list?
- Can another hospital or surgeon treat me sooner?
- If so, are they as good as you?
- Are there things I can do during my wait to make it easier?

## THINGS YOU CAN DO TO HELP

- Lobby provincial and federal governments to develop a system to manage waiting lists so the sickest are seen the soonest.
- Advocate that physicians and hospitals provide provincial governments with accurate, up-to-date information on waiting lists.

*Five*

# The Patient's Charter: Providing Care by the Clock

The sign on the wall at King's College Hospital says, "if you want to be seen, please take a ticket and the nurse will assess your turn." Like something out of a cheese store, patients in this London, England, hospital pull their numbered ticket from a red plastic dispenser in the emergency department. A large clock—like those found in grade schools—sits on a wall at the back of the room. Patients watch the big black hand tick minute by minute, waiting to see if the nurse calls them in five minutes, as she is supposed to under the Patient's Charter.

Triage nurse Lynn Burrough bellows out number sixty-two, sounding like a caller at a bingo hall. Clutching her ticket with the number sixty-two on it, Joyce Precieux walks in small steps towards the triage nurse, who assesses patients before sending them a doctor. Looking exhausted, Precieux, a delicate, soft-spoken woman in her sixtiess, tells Burrough that she has been sent to emergency by her general practitioner, after complaining to him of feeling faint. The anxiety in her voice is palpable. "It's terrible, I feel so faint all the time—it's hard to stand up," said Precieux in an interview during her wait. Obviously distraught over her condition, she hasn't a clue what could be wrong. But Precieux knows that the doctor's concern must have been substantial to send her to emergency. But what could it be?

Within four minutes, Precieux is assessed by Burrough and told to wait. After undergoing several tests that day, doctors tell Precieux she has an ulcer. She is prescribed Ranitidine tablets for one month. "The tablets seemed to work and I have had no problems since," she said almost a full year later. Afterwards, Precieux said she was very pleased with her care. "I felt my visit to the emergency unit was very satisfactory. I was taken good care of and although I was there a long time, this was due to the numerous tests the doctors had to undertake," she said. "This satisfied me as I felt my illness was being given serious attention."

Although true emergencies, those who have been shot, had a heart attack, or been hit by a car, are seen immediately by doctors, the bulk of patients who arrive in emergency wards turn out afterwards to not be serious cases. Still, prompt attention at emergency not only gives enormous consumer satisfaction, but it gives patients in Britain the comfort of knowing that government is tracking these waits and presumably will fix them when they become unwieldy. The tracking and publishing of waiting times is the hallmark of the Patient's Charter, a government-created set of national standards that culminates each year with the publication of hospital report cards in England, Scotland, and Wales.

Ambitious in scope, these ratings of hospitals by waiting lists began with former prime minister John Major. The simple premise was that you "should know what you're getting for your money and you should have sufficient information about where you'd like to be treated," said British Health Department spokesperson Richard Billinge in an interview in London, England. "Patients should know the waiting time in emergency, the waiting time for readmissions and cancelled operations."

And so, every year since 1994, patients have been able to see exactly how their local hospital measures up in fifty-nine different areas in which they can wait for care, be it in emergency, queuing for hip replacement surgery, or waiting for cardiac operations, in a publication entitled *The NHS Performance Guide,* in smaller regional guides, and even on CD-ROM. It's something no other country in the world has ever done.

Although consumer guides in the United States publish how many people die under the heart surgery scalpel by surgeon and by hospital, Great Britain has taken on what is probably the most complained about problem in its health care system—its waiting lists.

The "people pay all this money into the NHS [National

Health Service]. They ought to see how it is performing," said Billinge of what is informally referred to as league tables, government report cards that rate hospitals by how often they meet target times to see patients. Besides the five-minute target time in emergency, the Charter requires tracking of whether patients have been seen within one month of a last-minute cancellation of an operation and whether patients have been seen within thirteen weeks of a referral by a general practitioner, among others. "We thought we should have a yardstick to judge the best and worst hospitals."

The hospital report cards were desperately needed. England's hospitals were plagued by excessively long waits, and horror stories abounded of patients who died or lived in agony while waiting for care. The waiting lists also seemed to be unfair, as some waited only a few days while others queued for years.

When the government began publishing waiting lists in the early 1980s, there was "enormous variation. Depending on where you lived, you may wait three months or three years for a cataract operation or hip replacement," said Marianne Rigge, director of the College of Health, an advocacy group that tracks waiting lists and doctors' care. Rigge tells one story of a woman who waited two years for a hip replacement. Fearing she would miss the call, the elderly woman didn't even take a vacation. "She went shopping one afternoon and she missed the call [for the operation]. She had to wait another year," said Rigge.

The College of Health, largely funded by government,

essentially began as a service for patients looking for a hospital or physician who had a shorter waiting time. But that job has been largely overtaken by the Patient's Charter—one part of the much larger Citizen's Charter—which requires the rating of forty-two public services including hospitals, transportation, and education. All of these services are compared against national standards, which are published in annual "league tables."

Unlike Canada and every other country in the world, Great Britain actually tracks what the real waits are, and while patients are not given guarantees for care, the Patient's Charter does set targets and standards to which hospitals are expected to adhere. According to Stephen Dorrell, former secretary of state for health for the British government, there have been "dramatic improvements" in waiting times over the past few years, which is largely attributable to the publishing of performance charts and the government's funding commitment to reduce some of the very long waiting lists. Specifically, the "number of patients waiting more than two years for hospital admissions was 81,000 in March 1990. Today [1996], there are none and 18-month waits have been virtually eliminated," said Dorrell, who called the hospital report cards a "spur to action … . No one wants to be at the bottom and there is a great incentive to improve." In fact, the number of five-star performances of hospitals increased by twenty-three per cent from 1995 to 1996. Guy Howland, chief executive of the Patient's Association in England, a consumer advocacy group, stresses that the "real reason why the Charter is important is because it has raised awareness. People have seen the waiting lists come down a lot in recent years."

One hospital that has shortened its waiting lists quite substantially is King's College Hospital, a classic inner-city hospital catering to the rich of Dulwich Village and the struggling working class of nearby Camberwell. In 1994, sixty-eight per cent of patients waited thirty minutes or more for outpatient appointments with a specialist. Two years later, only ten per cent of patients waited longer than a half hour for their appointment with a specialist.

On the league tables or report cards, King's College Hospital had twenty-eight five-star ratings in 1995-96, which "put us at the top of the list with St. George's Hospital," said a proud Derek Smith, chief executive of King's College Hospital. Yet, the teaching hospital rated as "average" or only three stars on the league tables in emergency in the same year because it assessed patients within five minutes only eighty-eight per cent of the time. A downward arrow on the league table indicated that King's had a "significantly worse performance" compared to the year before.

Although patients can wait an awfully long time to see a doctor in the emergency ward, at least they are virtually guaranteed to be seen by a triage nurse, whose job it is to assess the severity of illness, something that's likely to be very reassuring to patients who may become very stressed as they wonder about the severity of their ailments. However, once assessed by a triage nurse, it can take hours to see a physician, depending on how many more severe cases there are in the emergency ward at that time. The government is proposing to deal with this, in part, by creating a new indicator to measure how many patients have to wait more than two hours to be admitted to a bed after going to emergency.

Simon Wood of the 870-bed King's College Hospital, notes that the Patient's Charter has "raised patient awareness and their expectations have increased. If you go and talk to GPs [general practitioners] they'll say 'patients are getting at me, demanding to be admitted to hospital.'" Aware of their rights, patients finally have some leverage to make demands. And Wood points out that there is a domino effect with the Patient's Charter: any service at King's College that receives less than three stars on the publicly released NHS performance or "league" tables must be reported to its board. In 1996, there were thirteen such areas, including general surgery, orthopedics, oral surgery, and dermatology.

Although the Charter has been deemed a success, "there are worries that the Patient's Charter is creating false expectations as they [patients] believe it's some form of guarantee," said Peter Ellis, former vice-president at Gemini Consulting in London. Dr. Stella Lowry of the British Medical Association agreed, saying while it's "important patients have information to use health services properly, it has its disadvantages."

David Knowles of the King's Fund, which promotes quality improvement in health through grants, policy analysis, and audit, calls the league tables "a bit of a joke. It ends up on the third page of the national newspapers—they're simplistic solutions." Smith doesn't believe the public cares much about the published hospital reports. "Who's interested in league tables? The press for about fifteen minutes, the NHS bureaucracy and government," he said.

Equally cynical about the hospital report cards was the late Maureen Dixon, then managing director of the London-based consulting firm Healthcare Risk Solutions Ltd. During an interview, Dixon said that league tables really don't give valuable information about how well a hospital performs surgery, because hospitals are measured only by how quickly they are able to see patients. "They don't tell you anything, but I do think the intention was very good," she said.

To dismiss the league tables as not telling a patient anything is harsh, as they actually tell patients quite a lot. For example, King's College Hospital admitted only one-third of patients for trauma and orthopedics such as hip and knee replacements within the target time of three months in 1995-96. But Eastbourne & County Healthcare in the same area matched that target almost three-quarters of the time, or seventy-two per cent, during the same time period. They may not tell patients how well the hospitals performed surgery, but the British government wants these types of report cards to be available in the future.

Like any system, the Patient's Charter isn't perfect and there will always be criticisms. But it's difficult to argue with a system that is not only effective but inexpensive—it costs less than a half million British pounds, or just over $1.2 million, to publish the league tables. Hospitals absorb the cost of tracking the waiting times as set out by the

Audit Commission, a watchdog body that is legislated to review the economy, efficiency, and effectiveness of the National Health Service.

Also, the Charter is in transition. Like anything revolutionary, it started with a measurement that was easy to gauge—waiting lists. By the next millennium, it aims to do clinical scorecards rating in which hospitals patients are most likely to suffer death and complications from medical procedures, though the procedures to be tracked have not yet been selected.

The bottom line, according to Billinge, is that "the public is very happy about it. And year by year, the overall performance of hospitals actually goes up. We always said we would start off in a small, manageable way. I guess a lot [of hospitals] aren't going to like the clinical scorecards either. If their [hospital] performance is poor, no one will want to go there."

Despite the effectiveness of the Patient's Charter in Great Britain, similar attempts to introduce one in Canada over the years have failed. A Patient's Bill of Rights was introduced in the Ontario Legislature by then Liberal Health Critic Elinor Caplan in the form of a private member's bill in April 1996. Bill 41 made it past second reading and was referred to committee with the simple aim to ensure patients received "appropriate and timely care." But it died without receiving final approval.

Alberta attempted to create a health charter in 1996 in what was to be a potential campaign plank for Premier Ralph Klein. Originally introduced at the Alberta

Progressive Conservative party convention in March 1996, the health charter was described by Klein to the media as a way to silence critics who charged the government was destroying medicare with its deep cuts. Months later, in a speech given on September 5, 1996, Klein said his government would introduce a draft health charter to foster "brutally honest" debate about acceptable waiting times for surgery or emergency services. It was at this speech that Klein made his very controversial remarks about self-inflicted illness when he stated, "Seventy per cent of people who go to a doctor or access the health care system are there because of something they have done to themselves."

At the time, Alberta Liberal health critic Howard Sapers believed those remarks signalled that the charter was going to be used as a tool to deinsure medically necessary services, which means they would no longer be covered under medicare. That, in turn, would force patients to dig deep into their pockets for health care. But an Alberta Health spokesperson denied the charter would be used in such a way.

One of the charter's authors, Alberta Member of the Legislature Dr. Lyle Oberg, said it would guarantee waiting lists for some surgeries would never go beyond the maximum clinically accepted time recommended by doctors. Oberg, chair of the government's standing committee on health restructuring, is seen by many to have been the "architect" of Alberta's health reform. Oberg said the health charter would likely apply to eight procedures, such as heart surgery, cataract removal, and joint replacement surgery. He expected the provincial government to fund it to the tune of about $5 million a year, which would reduce the waiting times in various areas. As Oberg saw it, the charter was to be an educational document, something that would explain the rights and responsibilities to those using the health care system.

In an article in the *Calgary Herald* on April 14, 1996, Oberg said he felt the charter would likely be legislated and backed by penalties against Regional Health Authorities that fail to comply with it. The key reason for the charter was to rationalize waiting lists by ensuring timely access to a list of medical procedures that currently have long queues. As well, it could be used as a guarantee to a certain level of access to health services no matter where one lived in the province. The charter was not without its critics, however. University of Alberta health economist Richard Plain dismissed it as a "public relations gimmick." To some, that suggested the charter wouldn't be objective and would be an attempt for the government to show what a good job it was doing, despite some deep cuts to the health care system.

Despite all the hype, delegates at the Alberta Progressive Conservative party's policy convention in September 1996 rejected the charter. There was concern about the cost required to potentially reduce waiting lists and the suggestion that patients could sue if they didn't get timely care. In the words of Linda Blumenthal, a delegate from Leduc, "the word 'charter' scares me. You end up in a very grey area of rights."

Federal Health Minister Alan Rock is interested in the idea of a Patient's Charter, or something similar that would inform patients of the standard of performance they should expect from the health care system. "I think it would be good if we had some mechanism by which we can both assess accountability in the system and reassure the public as to what they're entitled to expect," said Rock. "Any Charter of Rights or standards of accountability would have to be developed closely with the provinces. It's early yet. None of this is imminent." Although it's still in the idea stage, it appears the health minister is warming up to the idea of a report card on hospitals and waiting times.

Great Britain did what some have said could not be done: It tracked the waiting lists for many surgeries, doctors' appointments, and emergency waits in its hospitals and published them. Although some hospital presidents have grumbled about the extra work the tracking of waits has created, the Patient's Charter has helped whittle down some of the longer queues and allowed patients to shop for a hospital. Things aren't perfect: In December 1997, 974 patients waited longer than the eighteen-month Patient's Charter target for various procedures. Great Britain knows this number because they actually track their waiting lists. In most countries, the number on waiting lists is a mystery.

## QUESTIONS TO ASK YOUR POLITICIANS

- Why can't Canadians have a sytem that measures how long it takes to wait for surgeries and diagnostic tests?
- When will governments start to measure waiting lists?
- What do local and regional health authorities or provincial governments plan to do about some of the longer waiting lists, such as those for hip and knee replacements, for magnetic resonance imaging machines, or for cataract removal?

## THINGS YOU CAN DO TO HELP

- Lobby your provincial and federal governments to create a Patient's Charter of Rights.

*Six*

# The Pig and the Laparoscope

Like many strange stories, this one had a peculiar beginning. It started with a few pigs, a shiny new surgical wand, and doctors keen to learn a new operation that promised to revolutionize gall-bladder surgery. After general surgeons and some general practitioners in community hospitals spent a weekend or so operating on pigs, they went back to their hospitals and enthusiastically operated on patients. Some of these doctors had the benefit of more experienced surgeons to supervise them at their hospitals, but others did not.

Hospitals embraced the new surgery, medically known as laparoscopic cholecystectomy, in the late 1980s and in earnest in the early 1990s. Not only did it promise to be popular with patients because of its smaller scar and shorter recovery time, it could be a boon for hospital administrators who were keen to cut beds, trim budgets, and move more patients towards day surgery, thus keeping costs down.

Commonly called keyhole gall-bladder surgery, the procedure involves the use of a small fibre-optic scope, connected to a TV monitor, that allows the surgeon to use tiny instruments inside the body to excise unwanted tissue or organs. The operation is performed through four tubes inserted through holes in the abdomen. Excellent if done properly, the surgery cuts a potential five-day stay in hospital and six-inch scar down to a one- to two-day stay in hospital with four "keyhole-sized" scars, making it the ideal operation for patients who need their gall-bladders removed.

The surgery, complete with its new surgical gizmo, was first reported in 1987 by Phillipe Mouret of Lyon, France, and was picked up months later in the United States by Dr. Eddie Joe Reddick before making its way north to Canada. Five or six groups of general surgeons in Canada trained other general surgeons in the technique. During 1990-91, there were probably five to ten thousand laparoscopic cholecystectomies performed in Canada; in 1993-94, seventy-nine per cent of all gall-bladder removals were done by the new keyhole method.

Unfortunately, this surgery wasn't nearly as easy as it looked. It essentially transformed three dimensions into two, and while some doctors adapted to it well, others did not. Unlike most new surgeries, which are taught in teaching hospitals, this one began in community hospitals. Add uneven, sometimes poor, training to the mix and it was a recipe for trouble. "Some people took to it. Some guys thought it was no big deal," said Dr. Demetrius Litwin, who taught a course on how to perform the surgery when he worked at Toronto's Mount Sinai Hospital. "Other people did not. This is how the profession got fooled. They really didn't perceive it to be difficult."

But it was difficult, particularly for some surgeons whose only exposure to it was by performing it on animals. "Many people did [trained on] pigs. They would do two to six pigs in a weekend," Litwin said. But Litwin, who now works at the University of Massachusetts Medical Center, also found something else of concern. "A few GPs [general practitioners] who were practising in communities where they were doing open gall-bladder surgery wanted to learn how to do lap colies. This is a specialist procedure and they should not be doing it. The problem wasn't ill intentions so much as the failure to perceive there was a learning curve. I think most people did not realize they could be perceptibly fooled by the technology."

Along with the new operation and spotty training came the inevitable result of more complications to patients. Some patients suffered complications such as gastrointestinal problems; ailments in the stomach, intestines, and bladder; accidental punctures and lacerations; and a severed bile duct. (The bile duct carries bile from the liver to the gall-bladder and then to the duodenum, which is the beginning of the small intestine.) A severed or injured bile duct is marked by severe pain, fever, and jaundice as the bile juices spill into the patient's abdomen, causing an infection.

Worries about the speed at which the new surgery was being picked up were quickly noted in Canada, but they were not acted on. In January 1991, the Hospital Services Branch of Saskatchewan Health prepared a report for the province's Technology Advisory Committee, warning that "while the efficacy of the procedure has not been questioned, the safety of laparoscopic cholecystectomy has not yet been fully established," according to documents obtained under the Freedom of Information and Protection of Privacy Act. Saskatoon City Hospital was the first western hospital to perform the procedure in 1990, and in that year performed more than 150 cases.

The Saskatchewan report cautioned that keyhole gallbladder surgery was being "diffused,"or picked up too rapidly, by hospitals without a proper evaluation. "Isolated cases of injury to adjacent organs have occurred but the frequency and severity of these complications are not known," the report said. "There is some controversy within the medical profession respecting how rapidly this technique should be allowed to diffuse prior to receiving the results of more thorough evaluations of the procedure." Despite that 1991 warning, it appears nothing was done.

The Canadian Association of General Surgeons also had concerns around the same time and chose to deal with them by drafting a policy on who should perform the surgery. Signed by Dr. Ronald B. Passi, the chair of the association's subcommittee on endoscopy, it stated that not only should the surgery be located in university centres but those learning how to do it must perform the procedure on humans. Traditionally, surgeries are pioneered in teaching centres and doctors are trained not only on animals but assist more senior surgeons on real human patients before moving on to do the surgery unassisted. As well, only general surgeons experienced with the traditional open gall-bladder removals and the management of its complications should perform the surgery, the report said. Since these were only guidelines, there was no way to enforce them.

Unlike the technology of the laparoscope, which was evaluated by the Canadian Medical Devices Bureau, the new procedure was not monitored by a government or hospital body. Not then and not now. That's because doctors are considered to be "independent" physicians who work out of hospitals, and it is up to their professional bodies and hospitals to ensure that training is adequate.

But this story is not just about keyhole gall-bladder surgery. It's about how a new technology and surgical procedure swept through hospital operating rooms like a prairie fire on a dry August day with no regulations, no watchdog, and few standards. It happened with gall-bladders, and it is happening to a lesser extent with hysterectomies and hernia and cancer surgery as the laparoscope is used in those operations. The laparoscope is the shining example of what happens when there is no formal body to monitor and evaluate the use of the pair of hands using a new technology.

Just as Transport Canada wouldn't allow a pilot to fly a new aircraft a couple of times and then take up hundreds of people on it, so the regulating bodies should not allow surgeons to pick up a new surgical technique and work out their learning curve on patients without first being monitored and evaluated. Transport Canada checks out pilots who move to newer planes, yet no such regulatory body does the equivalent with surgeons or doctors learning new procedures or operations. Allowing surgeons to work out their learning curves on patients as they did with this new gall-bladder surgery is akin to suggesting it's permissible if a few planeloads of passengers crash until the pilot gets a feel for the new airplane controls.

And if the United States was any indication, there were reasons for Canadians to be concerned early on that there was a problem, not with the laparoscope but with the surgeons using it. In the United States, reports of patients suffering sliced bile ducts, lacerated livers, perforated bowels and bladders, cut blood vessels, and bile leaks began to surface to an extent that doctors had never observed with the traditional, open surgery. "The incidence of major bile duct injury may have increased at least thirty-fivefold and the introduction of this new technique has resulted in injuries in great vessels and organs rarely or never reported before," said Dr. Harvey Bernard, chief surgical advisor for the New York State Department of Health. In the early 1990s, hospitals were "either negligent or uninformed about the requirements to report this."

Quickly, a doctor's professional body, the Society of American Gastrointestinal Endoscopic Surgeons, put out its own warning label, stating that doctors should have received credentials in diagnostic laparoscopy before doing the operation. As well, the society stated that the surgeon's training director should put in writing the training, experience, and observed competency of the doctor. "Attendance at short courses which do not provide supervised hands-on training is not an acceptable substitute for the development of equivalent competency," it said. It noted that doctors performing the surgery should be monitored through existing quality assurance programs in hospitals.

Tough-minded medical officials in New York State also felt it important to act. They warned the public of the dangers of the surgery by setting up a hotline in 1992, specifically for Medicare and Medicaid patients, which are a mix of those who are elderly and who receive government assistance. "We felt we had to. At the time this procedure wasn't credentialled in any way. As a consequence, there were very high death rates," said Dr. Pascal Imperato, medical director of research, development, and epidemiology for the Island Peer Review Organization (IPRO), a state-financed Medicare peer review group that tracks the use of health care services.

Trained as nurses, the New York State hotline operators urged patients to find out if the surgeon was formally trained in a recognized program in laparoscopic cholecystectomy, if the surgeon was board-certified, the number of operations the surgeon had performed, and what his or her complication rates were. "We want patients to be partners in their health care—not victims of it," said nurse Sheila McCullagh, director of consumer relations at IPRO.

In addition to injuries, Americans were also seeing another problem: the suggestion that too many gall-bladders were being removed, with the state of Pennsylvania reporting a fifty-two per cent increase. There were similar increases in Canada, which prior to the early 1990s had the highest rate of gall-bladder removal in the world and then saw its rate climb even further with the use of the laparoscope. About seventy-two thousand of these operations are done in Canada every year. But just because patients have gallstones doesn't mean they need surgery. Although gallstones can cause infection, severe pain, and several other complications, many people with them have no symptoms at all and merely need to change their diet.

In Canada, surgeons who repaired severed bile ducts—once a very infrequent injury—were now seeing more patients needing these serious repairs in their operating rooms, the direct result of patients undergoing gall-bladder surgery. As well, more patients were being sent back to Ontario hospitals with gastrointestinal problems, including ailments in the stomach, intestines, and gall-bladder, following the surgery.

There were also concerns among surgeons that some of their colleagues weren't performing enough of the operations to maintain their skills. "When the operation was initiated, people used to say you had to do ten or fifteen to be good at it. Maybe today, you have to do at least fifty. Now, it would be fair to say you need to be doing a lot—thirty to forty a year," said Dr. Sherif Hanna, a surgeon at North York's Sunnybrook Health Science Centre.

In 1992, when the surgery was still relatively new, Michelle Miles went to a hospital in Kitchener, Ontario, to get her gall-bladder removed by Dr. David Judges, but what transpired in that operating room would change her life for ever. Using a method he had only used twice before, Judges inadvertently sliced through the veins near Miles's spine, causing profuse bleeding. Despite attempts by another surgeon to repair those cuts, Miles was left brain-damaged from what was supposed to be a routine operation on a fit woman in her early twenties.

Miles sued Judges, and at the trial experts testified she had suffered an extremely extensive and massive stroke, with a "large area of death on the left side of the brain," according to the sixty-nine-page judgment written by Justice Paul G. Philp. Consequently, Miles suffers from significant speech, visual, and comprehension impairment, and experts say she will never be able to work or support herself again. Six months after the injury, Miles's condition had barely improved. She will never be able to go back to her $16,000-a-year job as a polishing-machine operator at KW Optical Company, nor will she likely ever work again. The dream of going back to school for a career in early childhood education was dead, as was the hope that she could be a full mother to her little girl, Connie. Nor can she indulge in such hobbies as knitting, fishing, reading a book, or watching a television program. Gone not only is her health but any hope of having a career or any semblance of a normal life. She has a poverty of words, but she got her point across when she testified: "Brain gone big time."

At the civil trial, Miles took the stand to testify about the injury, and "while she looked quite normal and attractive, when you listen to her and interview her, you realize that there are problems in her intellectual and cognitive abilities as well as physical problems," Philp wrote. Miles's restricted speech is called Broca's aphasia, caused by damage to the portion of her brain responsible for motor speech. She also suffers from receptive aphasia, which is the loss of the ability to easily and completely understand spoken words.

Although Miles is able to write in an awkward manner, a sampling of her writing entered as evidence at the trial looked to the judge to be done by someone in grade two. As Philp noted, "the twelve partial sentences that she wrote took her two hours and twenty minutes to complete."

At the trial, Judges was unable to give any explanation as to why this injury happened. "He did not know why this injury happened but denied that it was from lack of care or skill," according to the judgment. However, the slashed blood vessels were about twelve inches from where the operation to remove the gall-bladder was being performed. "While Dr. Judges may not have had the experience of his fellow surgeons, he has held himself out to Ms. Miles that he possesses that degree of skill of the average general surgeon in his community in the use of a direct trocar insertion," wrote Philp.

Although Judges had performed about twenty keyhole gall-bladder surgeries, he had performed only two using what is called a "trocar direct insertion," which is potentially riskier than the "Veres" needle technique. Philp noted that Judges "should have told his patient that he had only performed two trocar direct insertions and that his assistant ... was more experienced than he." That was important, as Miles "should have been given the opportunity of requesting the services of a more experienced surgeon in the use of the trocar direct insertion technique or he [Judges] should have used the "Veres" needle technique with which he was much more experienced."

There were two major techniques used to perform the surgery. One involved the direct insertion of a ten-millimetre tube called a trocar, which was about ten inches long, just below the belly button. It was inserted on a forty-five-degree angle downwards through the layers of the abdominal wall and into the abdominal cavity. When the trocar is in place, the blade is removed and a laparoscope, or camera, is inserted into the hollow tube. This enables surgeons to see on a screen the abdominal cavity and various organs including the gall-bladder, which is located below the bottom of the ribcage on the right-hand side, behind the liver. After that, two more trocars, about half the diameter of the major trocar, are used to insert other instruments that are used to cut and remove the gall-bladder through another ten-millimetre trocar.

The tip of the trocar consists of a sharp, triangular, spear-shaped knife that cuts through the abdominal wall, which is made up of layers of skin, fat, fascia or muscle, and the peritoneum. When the trocar reaches the abdomen and resistance lessens, the knife retracts and is replaced automatically by a plastic shield. This plastic shield clicks into position as soon as the resistance felt by the layers of the abdominal wall disappears, which prevents the knife from cutting an organ.

Another technique, preferred by many surgeons teaching keyhole gall-bladder surgery, involved the insertion of a thin, sharp "Veres" needle into the abdomen. There, it would inflate the abdomen with carbon dioxide to create a larger space or safety zone between the abdominal wall and underlying structures. Called insufflation, the procedure created a larger area between the abdominal wall and the abdominal cavity—or a "safer" area for arrival of the trocar. The trocar was then inserted through the wall into the abdominal cavity. Ideally, the gall-bladder was pulled through the abdominal incision and disposed of.

Philp had to decide whether the injuries Miles suffered were due to medical misadventure, an "error in judgement," or negligence. In the end, Philp found Judges' "negligence was the cause of brain damage suffered by Ms. Miles" in a May 1997 decision. The damages amounted to about $2.1 million, said lawyer Ron Manes, who acted for Miles.

Miles was one of many who began legal proceedings against their doctors for injuries sustained during the procedure. Dr. André Duranceau, who is on the Executive Committee of the Canadian Medical Protective Association, the doctors' defence fund, said lawsuits are up. In the last twenty years, there were fifty-eight lawsuits due to bile duct injuries during open gall-bladder operations but over a six-year period (1991-97) 175 lawsuits have been started for laparoscopic surgeries. Some of them involve bile duct injuries, cut vessels, and blood in the chest cavity.

Duranceau said he is not certain why the number of law-suits is up, but notes laparoscopic surgery is being done more than ever and not just on the gall-bladder.

Some patients had complications but decided not to sue. One of them, Toronto psychologist Miriam Rosin, was wounded during her operation by a surgeon who told her he had performed fifty of the procedures in 1990. "He was-n't a confident person—there was something pathetic about him. I took pity on him and I think that's why I let him operate on me. I know I shouldn't think like that, I'm a psy-chologist. When I came to, he said he'd nicked my liver. I was home the next day." Two days later, Rosin, who was sixty-nine at the time, was rushed to emergency with a high temperature and stomach cramps—a direct result of the so-called "nick." She was in the hospital for sixteen days with a tube in her abdomen to drain the infection in her belly.

Linda Shay's experience with gall-bladder surgery not only left her ill but ruined her financially. Shay was a Master's student at Dalhousie University in Halifax and a single mother of four working part-time when she learned she needed her gall-bladder removed. In anticipation of her December 1991 surgery, she took time off work, but there was a problem at the hospital. Shay was told the sur-geon scheduled to do the operation had had his operating privileges suspended, so he couldn't perform the opera-tion. "The only option presented to me was to have the remaining surgeon with privileges do the surgery," said Shay of the small-town Nova Scotia hospital. Although she had a "bad" feeling about it, Shay "reluctantly agreed."

Immediately after the operation, Shay experienced severe pain. It took a month to diagnose the medical mystery, but doctors figured it out: Shay's bile duct had been severed. She was told that most of her bile duct had been removed during the operation. She was sent away to have a Roux-en-Y operation, which means doctors had to reconstruct a bile duct with remaining tissue. Of all the reconstructive surgeries for cut bile ducts, surgeons say the Roux-en-Y has the worst outcome. Doctors do it only when there is little of the bile duct left.

Despite surgeries and other treatments, Shay initially felt better, but that feeling didn't last long. What was supposed to be a routine gall-bladder removal changed Shay's life for ever. "I lost my schooling, I was off work for months during which time I had no medical insurance coverage [drug coverage], I lost my home, I am ruined financially, and I am unwell most of the time," said Shay. "I am on medication for symptomatic relief."

And there were others. Louis Juhasz of Haliburton had the gall-bladder surgery at an Ontario hospital in November 1996, but less than a week after he was discharged from the hospital he was rushed back with "severe abdominal pain." Doctors told him his "bile duct had burst open." Juhasz was in the hospital for three more weeks, only to be readmitted once again for jaundice. "They inserted a biliary drainage tube," wrote Juhasz, then later a stent, and then a catheter for two months. "I hope you can use my example and help other people to be alert about the possibility of surgery," he wrote. "I am a sixty-eight-year-old man who was and hopefully will be [a] very healthy, active person."

Dorothy Gordon of Ottawa had surgery in the summer of 1996. Shortly after, she experienced discharge from one of the incisions and was in pain up until Thanksgiving of 1996. "A few small pieces of a gallstone emerged [from the incision] and I suspect there are a few slivers left. As you can imagine, it has been a rotten year and I wonder whether this discharge will go on for ever," she wrote in a letter. "Prior to this operation, I had been in excellent health despite being seventy-two."

Spilled gall-bladder stones—not a common problem with the open gall-bladder operation—were being reported as surgeons using the laparoscope were inadvertently puncturing the gall-bladder while trying to remove it. Although some suggested this puncturing of the gall-bladder was an incidental occurrence that didn't affect patients, researchers in Vancouver found otherwise. In a *Canadian Journal of Surgery* study, Drs. Emma Patterson and Alexander Nagy said bile and gallstone spillage occurred in thirty-two to forty per cent of keyhole procedures. While spilled stones are easy to mop up with the open procedure, it is far more difficult with the closed, keyhole operation. The doctors estimated that stones are left in patients' bodies thirteen to thirty-two per cent of the time with the keyhole operation. "Surgeons don't think this is a problem because they have been taught it's not a problem," Nagy said afterwards in an interview. "But I have four legal cases sitting on my desk involving patients injured by spilled gall-bladder stones." Other studies have noted that these spilled stones can obstruct the bowel, migrate to the ovaries or the chest, and even prompt the development of an abscess. Some stones do nothing and sit in the body, but it isn't worth leaving them in a patient to find out if they'll have an adverse effect.

The first Canadian study that set out to track complications, bile duct injuries and readmission to hospital was published in the *Canadian Medical Association Journal.* Written by Dr. Marsha Cohen and Wendy Young, the peer-reviewed study was the first in Canada to focus on injuries that occurred during keyhole gall-bladder operations in Ontario from 1989 to 1994. It found the bile duct injury rate had increased by 305 per cent for all gall-bladder surgeries. It found the number of patients readmitted to hospital within thirty days of receiving keyhole gall-bladder surgery had doubled during that time and that Ontario had an overall one per cent bile duct injury rate. That means for every one hundred patients getting the operation, one of them had a bile duct injury.

In the early 1990s, there were also indications that surgeons were having a tough time with the operation. In one Ontario hospital, a surgeon had to convert from the closed gall-bladder operation to the open one half of the time. Three other hospitals had conversion rates of more than twenty per cent, which means they had to abandon the laparoscopic operation in favour of the open one at least one-fifth of the time, according to Cohen's second peer-reviewed study published in the Institute for Clinical

Evaluative Sciences in Ontario's (ICES) *Practice Atlas* publication. Elsewhere, a study in the *Atlas* stated, "we found no relationship between a hospital's rate of bile duct injury and its rate of conversion to open procedures." The same report showed unnamed hospitals with bile duct injury rates of eight and ten per cent.

Apparently concerned about the high reporting of injuries, scientists in the publication wrote: "We recommend that physicians participate in the monitoring of hospital-specific mortality rates, bile duct injury rates, and indications for cholecystectomy as part of quality assurance and risk management activities." Still, ICES researchers didn't name the hospitals, mostly because these institutions did low numbers of operations, which one would think was a problem in itself. But according to Dr. David Naylor, then chief executive officer of the Institute for Clinical Evaluative Sciences in Ontario, he was very concerned about "potentially doing damage to the reputation of perfectly good colleagues." Cohen suggested to Naylor that a chart audit should be done of hospitals that reported high injury rates so researchers could confirm the precise number of injuries and exactly how severe they were. In a chart audit, surgeons or other doctors pore over the medical charts to find out exactly what was wrong. Cohen's suggestion was refused.

The real problem with the keyhole gall-bladder surgery is that there is "no credentialling. Anybody can do it. You see one, do one, and then teach one," said Cohen afterwards. There are also "no surveillance mechanisms and no mechanisms to ensure the credentialling of surgeons," she said. And therein lies a great irony. While there is little control over introducing new surgeries and technologies to doctors in Canada, there are very stringent protocols established for the release of new drugs in this country. While the Health Protection Branch of Health Canada makes pharmaceutical companies prove that new drugs not only work but don't do any harm, there is nothing comparable for surgeons and new procedures.

Cohen's scientific papers received a fair amount of publicity, including newspaper stories and a segment on CBC's *The Health Show.* Of great concern was the fact that the hospitals that appeared to have high bile duct injury rates were unidentified, leaving prospective patients unable to protect themselves. The public needed protecting, yet there seemed to be no one who was willing to do it.

I made a request under the Freedom to Information and Protection of Privacy Act in late fall 1997, requesting the names of hospitals and their bile duct injury rates over a five-year period. The documents indicated that 156 hospitals had reported 938 bile duct injuries to the Canadian Institute for Health Information over a five-year period. Hospitals are required by law to report on patients' discharges what operations they received, their complications, and the length of their stay. Hospitals reported those injuries from 1990, when the procedure began in earnest, until 1995-96, the latest data available.

When Cohen was shown the most recent data, she called them a "red flag for further investigation." If anything, she thought the figures could be conservative, as they didn't include patients who were injured, then sent to a tertiary care centre to have reconstructive surgery.

But when the data were published a third time, it wasn't in a scientific journal that the profession could easily ignore but in articles I wrote for the *Toronto Star*, the largest-circulation daily in Canada, complete with a chart of twenty-one hospitals that were identified, using Cohen's method, as having above-average to high bile duct injury rates. There was a lot of controversy over the figures, and three surgeons at one hospital filed a lawsuit for libel against the *Star*. The surgeons say there were no bile duct injuries during the five-year period. Indeed, an independent review of the charts at that hospital afterwards indicated there were no bile duct injuries. The lawsuit singled out myself and Don Sellar, the ombudsman, who had done an investigation of the journalism, and wrote in a column: "Clearly Priest used the best available data to raise an accountability issue and a question: Without independent audits of hospital charts, how are patients to make informed choices about where to have gall-bladder surgery?"

As part of that controversy, hospitals disputed the figures, claiming Cohen's methodology was flawed and offering revised figures of their own. But it would be a later scientific study published in the *Canadian Medical Association Journal* that would suggest there was a problem with the way hospitals coded their injuries. In this study, Dr. Bryce Taylor, a University of Toronto professor of surgery who specializes in biliary tract operations, scrutinized some medical records made available by eighteen of the twenty-one hospitals named in the *Star* article. He found the data system tracking injuries suffered by patients having gall-bladder surgery to be vague and confusing and recommended it be revamped. Later he told *Star* medical reporter Leslie Papp: "The recording of these things is really flawed."

Of the 104 medical records identified by Cohen's method and submitted for review, Taylor found only twenty-eight had complications that were considered "clinically relevant." Although he concludes the incidence of major bile duct injury following keyhole gall-bladder surgery in Ontario is "unclear," his research indicates it is far less than what Cohen had suggested.

The major limitation of Taylor's study was that hospitals were not only able to select their own charts, they weren't given detailed instructions on exactly how that should be done. Taylor noted that it is "possible that they did not select the records randomly and may have held back records that revealed complications that I would have classed as clinically relevant." During the review, two questions popped up. Why did hospitals code clinically irrelevant injuries? And was there a financial advantage for hospitals to do this? Taylor didn't answer these questions.

After reading Taylor's study, Dr. Vivek Goel, lead editor of the ICES *Practice Atlas*, who had published the research pointing out high bile duct injury rates, issued a carefully worded news release. Down in the second-last paragraph,

Goel said Taylor's findings "invalidate the sections of the *Atlas* that allude to bile duct injuries."

This is all very confusing to the public. Two scientific studies suggest there are a lot of injuries occurring at hospitals, yet the latest one suggests the coding of those injuries cannot be relied on and the injuries likely aren't any higher than with the previous open method of removing gall-bladders. This kind of contradiction is not unusual, as science tends to be a series of building blocks and researchers have a tendency to find what they start out looking for.

However, it does leave the public with the unsettling feeling of not knowing whom and what they should believe. Despite the contradictory studies, patients are left with an identical problem: They have little information on how to select a hospital to get their gall-bladder surgeries. And no one has come forward to do a thorough, comprehensive investigation of all hospitals providing the surgery by looking at their medical charts and coding practices.

What patients do know is this: The training for this procedure was uneven, ranging from poor to excellent depending on the hospital; there was and still is no regulatory body that ensures that the hands using new technologies are skilled; and some patients were the victim of surgeons' learning curves. However, Dr. Litwin, the surgeon who taught others on the laparoscope, says training is excellent now and the procedure is very safe.

It's ludicrous to not have a regulatory body watch over the training of the pair of hands using a new technology. Nowhere else in society would that be acceptable. Can you imagine a car manufacturer trying to argue that it took a while for the engineers to get the hang of creating a new car design and it was acceptable to work out the learning curve in the form of a few automobile crashes? Or that a few subway crashes were acceptable until a new driver got used to a change in technology? It's insane, but that is exactly what some would have you believe is acceptable medical practice.

Scientists, too, hide behind their anonymous data, often not willing to point the finger at hospitals and content to have their publications printed in leading medical journals, where no hard questions are asked. Naming hospitals with injury and complication rates would not only be safer for members of the public, it would ensure that the research is far more rigorously analysed and peer-reviewed before being published in medical journals.

As Dr. Ken Bassett of the British Columbia Office on Health Technology Assessment pointed out, "The provinces have to step in and make hospitals, and therefore surgeons, more accountable. The question is: Who should report it?"

## QUESTIONS TO ASK

*Culled from a number of experts, the following are a few questions to ask before getting keyhole gall-bladder surgery.*

- Do I really need this procedure?
- Is there another way to treat gall-bladder disease, such as medical therapy, change of diet, or watchful waiting? (Just because one has gallstones doesn't mean that the gall-bladder has to be removed. Nor does one attack necessarily mean the patient is guaranteed a second.)
- If the answer is yes to surgery, ask for the bile duct injury rates and accidental puncture rates by surgeon.
- How many procedures have you done alone, not just assisted on? If the surgeon is reluctant to answer this very important question, look elsewhere. A doctor who can't defend his or her abilities probably isn't the right surgeon for you.
- Are bile duct injuries and accidental punctures reviewed with individual surgeons? If the answer is yes, chances are the hospital is keeping a watchful eye on the quality of the procedures.
- Trust your instincts. If a surgeon doesn't feel right, no matter what his or her "statistics" are, don't let him or her operate on you. You are picking up on something–listen to it.

## THINGS YOU CAN DO TO HELP

- Demand that the provincial and federal governments ensure

physicians and other staff are adequately trained in the safe and appropriate use of new technologies.

- Demand that hospitals monitor the use of new technologies and restrict the privileges of physicians who do not show high levels of competence.

## *Seven*

# Silent Knife

If you live in Ontario, you are twice as likely to receive coronary artery bypass graft surgery and angioplasty as someone living in England. But still, half as likely as an American.

A pregnant woman is more than one-and-a-half times as likely to have a Caesarean section if she lives in British Columbia than if she lives in Manitoba or Alberta.

And when it comes to hysterectomies, Nipissing/Timiskaming is tops in the province in Ontario, with surgeons in that area removing the uteruses of women more than two-and-a-half times as often as doctors do in Toronto, the city with the lowest hysterectomy rate in Ontario.

Ontario men fifty and older with prostate cancer, the most common cancer affecting men, are most likely to get radical prostate surgery if they live in the Wellington-Dufferin region and least likely if they reside in Algoma, which has one-sixth of the top region's rate.

And Canada removes more gall-bladders per capita than anywhere else, even though its citizens do not suffer proportionately more gall-bladder-disease.

What does this all mean?

To some, it suggests too much—or maybe too little—surgery is being performed on patients in Canada. Some scientists believe that while some of these surgeries—such as hysterectomies, tonsil removals, radical prostate surgeries, and gall-bladder operations—are being done too often, it's difficult to say which rate of surgery is right.

For example, when it comes to cardiac artery bypass graft surgery and angioplasty, a nonsurgical procedure that improves blood flow to the heart, Canadians have twice as many as those in the United Kingdom. Specifically, Canadians received 104 of the procedures per 100,000 people, according to 1991 figures published in the *Canadian Journal of Cardiology*. Those in the U.K. received 52 per 100,000, while Americans got the most with 268 per 100,000, according to 1992 figures published in *Heart*.

"It should be understood that high and low rates of surgery don't necessarily correspond to more or less appropriate use of surgery," said Dr. David Naylor, then chief executive officer of the government-funded Institute for Clinical Evaluative Sciences in Ontario, which tracks the use of health care services in that province. Exceptions include hysterectomies, "where in some regions we may well be overutilizing a procedure that can frequently be avoided," and hip and knee replacement surgeries, where "we are in general underutilizing those procedures in the low rate area."

But Canadians could learn a thing or two from U.S. scientists, who don't want information about the different rates of surgeries by area to stay within the elite circles of doctors who may—or may not—pay attention to them. Dr. John Wennberg, director of Dartmouth University's Center for the Evaluative Clinical Sciences in Hanover, New Hampshire, has been successful at getting these differing surgery rates out to the public. He does it for this reason: there is so much uncertainty in medicine and such striking differences in the rate of operations by region, the public should know if they're living in a surgical hotspot so they can make informed decisions on whether to get surgery.

"It's one thing for policymakers to suggest that local citizens best understand local needs. It's quite a leap—and a dangerous one at that—to permit wide variations in virtually every part of the health care system, while there is no evidence that patients are the source of the variations or that more expenditures lead to better health care," said Wennberg. Three decades ago, with colleague Alan Gittelsohn, he pioneered what is commonly called small area variations, a scientific term to explain the differences in surgery rates by region or county. In that time, he has made interactive video discs to help patients make informed health care choices, he has helped push the U.S. Congress into funding research to reduce the large number of inappropriate surgeries in some regions, and he has improved the quality of care south of the border.

When Wennberg's *Dartmouth Atlas of Health Care in the United States* was released in spring 1996, Dick Davidson, president of the American Hospital Association, pointed out that, "In the end, real reform of the health system can be achieved only when individuals can make informed decisions about their care and become more accountable for their health." The *Dartmouth Atlas*, which is the product of ten years of research and is produced by the American Hospital Association, found that physician and hospital preferences—not patient preferences or needs—have resulted in the variation of services provided to those south of the border.

Whether a woman receives a mastectomy or breast-conserving surgery for cancer, for example, depends on where she lives and where her doctor was trained. Rates of radical prostate surgery are 3.7 times higher in Salt Lake City, Utah, than in Louisville, Kentucky. And patients are twice as likely to get coronary artery bypass graft surgery in Birmingham, Alabama; Little Rock, Arkansas; and Dayton, Ohio, than they are in the Bronx, Honolulu, and Denver regions. Looking for the back surgery capital of America? It's Provo, Utah.

"The regional editions of the *Atlas* raise the question again, 'What is the "right" rate of use of medical care?'" asked Wennberg, lead researcher on the *Atlas* project. "It's not that patients in areas with lower coronary artery bypass procedure rates are going without treatment, but that they are being treated with other approaches—medical instead of surgical management of angina, for example. We won't know which rate is the right one until we let patients choose according to their own preferences."

Like Canada, the Americans realize there will always be

some difference in the amount of surgery performed from one area to another, but if there are very large differences, U.S. researchers are far more aggressive in tracking down the problem with an eye to protecting the public. Despite their strong stance of individualism, Americans have a much better record than Canada of protecting and informing the public when it comes to regulating, studying, and monitoring their health care system.

In Canada, although researchers publish the large differences in surgery rates, there is rarely the follow-through there is in the United States. The reason may be our reluctance to seem accusatory or simply the fact that some are resistant to saying that it is the surgeons' problem. "In many instances, quality problems have probably less to do with the individual practitioner and much more to do with the way we organize our health care system," said Naylor, who has spent years studying the differences in surgery rates by region and hospital.

Much of the Canadian research has been published in academic journals, and is written in language inaccessible to the average reader. Consequently, the public rarely finds out about these problems of too much or too little surgery in the areas that they live. And yet this information is relevant to those facing surgery. For example, if you were a woman living in an area that removed uteruses three times more than another region, you might be more likely to question the need for a hysterectomy, particularly if you had fibroids or abnormal bleeding, conditions that can often be managed with medication.

Others who might like to know the rates of surgery for their area or hospital include pregnant women not keen to have a Caesarean section or episiotomy; patients who have suffered a gall-bladder attack; mothers whose children have sore throats or infected tonsils; or those with breast cancer who need to choose between breast-conserving surgery and a mastectomy. For these and other people facing surgery as an option, comparisons are needed to find out if they live in a Canadian region deemed a surgical hotspot.

Internist Dr. Eugene Vayda, who has published studies on surgical variation rates across Canada, found that the removal of tonsils and adenoids had the greatest variation of any of the thirty-nine surgical procedures he studied across Canada between April 1, 1988, and March 31, 1990. As one of the most common operations performed on children, the medical indications for when to operate has garnered a fair amount of controversy. Others on Vayda's top ten list of surgical variability include extraction of lens [cataract surgery] (2); tonsillectomy without adenoidectomy (3); hysterectomy (4); excision of (semilunar) cartilage of knee (5); Caesarean section (6); excision of intervetebral disc (7); adenoidectomy without tonsillectomy (8) gall-bladder removal (9); and radical prostate surgery or prostatectomy (10). Operations at the very bottom of the scale—where there was little variation—include kidney transplants, repair of a hole in the heart, kidney removal, an operation to remove the spleen, the excision of brain tissue, heart valve surgery, radical mastectomy, amputation of lower limb, and resection of the large bowel.

Medicine will always be uncertain, and we may never be able to say for certain why some rates are higher than others. But patients aren't trying to solve a scientific puzzle; they are trying to get the best health care available and that can only be done if they give informed consent. And what may not be good enough data for some scientists can be overwhelmingly enough information for a health care consumer.

When Canadian surgical variation rates, particularly for hysterectomies, are published, the response from general surgeons is depressingly familiar. They charge first that data are flawed, usually basing this assertion on their own personal experience of being a good doctor and not performing unnecessary operations. Many state that patients are driving up the need for surgery, as if somehow a stampede of people want to go under the knife in Canada's hospitals, especially women demanding that their uteruses be removed. A similar reaction has been observed with higher Caesarean section rates as surgeons justify it as a way to keep infant death rates down, even though other countries with much lower Caesarean section rates have equally healthy babies and moms.

"Some surgeons' groups are quite gracious," said Vayda. "But there are other groups who think that I'm out of my mind and it's beneath discussion, beneath their dignity" to talk about the differences in surgical rates by region or census division. That's why he believes it is crucial for the public to have access to the information. "I think taking the data and bringing it into public consciousness is important. I hope to change [doctors'] behaviour that way."

•

The one operation that has captured probably more attention than any other is hysterectomies, largely because the differences in surgical rates are so stark. It is the most frequently performed gynecological operation in Canada, with just shy of sixty thousand performed each year. A hysterectomy, which can be performed abdominally or vaginally, can be done by removing the womb with or without the cervix. Some are even performed with a laparoscope in what is commonly called keyhole surgery because of its small incisions.

While a hysterectomy is a definite must for those who have uterine cancer, some researchers believe they are done far too often on women with abnormal bleeding, fibroids, and prolapse of the uterus (this is when the uterus descends from its normal position). Other reasons women have hysterectomies include cancer of the cervix, ovaries, or fallopian tubes and endometriosis, a condition in which pieces of womb lining grow outside the uterus.

Depending on where a woman lives, she is far more likely to have her uterus removed, or as some have jokingly remarked, be cleaned out like a junk drawer, before she reaches menopause. In fact, in Vayda's 1996 study of variation rates of thirty-nine surgical procedures performed in Canada, hysterectomy ranked as the operation with the fourth *most* variation. By that, researchers mean that from one area to another, the rate of surgery varied dramatically—something that can't be explained by the illness of patients alone. "The fourth most variable procedure, hysterectomy, exhibits truly high underlying variability in rates across Canada," wrote study authors Jane Gentleman and Vayda in the *Canadian Medical Association Journal*. "This procedure also yielded the highest number of outliers (twenty-six); of these, eighteen were at the high end of the distribution and eight were at the low end." By outliers, they mean there were surgeons in areas who did far more—or far fewer—hysterectomies than doctors in the rest of the country.

"Until better outpatient surgery data are available, recommendations regarding operations performed in large numbers on an outpatient basis cannot be made. However, the provinces could, for example, turn their attention to cholecystectomy, prostatectomy, hysterectomy, intervertebral disc (back) surgery, and Caesarean section," wrote the authors. They are politely asking those with authority to look more closely at the high and differing rates of these surgeries. Gentleman and Vayda concluded: "If, as we suspect, the high surgical procedure rates are too high, then steps taken to reduce the rates will improve health and the quality of life while saving tax dollars."

After the research was published, there was disagreement on just what conclusions one could draw from Gentleman's and Vayda's study. Entitled "Quill on Scalpel," Drs. Ved Tandan and Bernard Langer wrote in the *Canadian Medical Association Journal* that although the article was interesting, "it is more useful as background material for developing a hypothesis than for drawing conclusions or making recommendations." The duo said that "it is not the rate of performance of a surgical procedure but the outcome on the health of the population that is important."

Suggestions that research should really look at the "outcome" instead of the differing rates of surgeries isn't a very useful one. For example, if a hysterectomy was a success in that the operation helped control a woman's bleeding, that would be a good outcome. But if she didn't need the operation in the first place and could have been treated just as well with drugs without the risk of surgery, then it doesn't much matter that the operation was a success, does it? While the outcome for surgery may be a good one, that doesn't say anything about whether the surgeon should do the operation in the first place.

And it's not as if once a woman gets her uterus removed, the hassle of related health problems are over. The rates of complications range from twenty-four per cent for the vaginal type of surgery to forty-three per cent for the abdominal ones, of which post-operative fever and infection account for the majority of complications. As well, patients should also be forewarned about the risk of hemorrhage and damage to surrounding organs.

Nora Coffey, director of Hysterectomy Education Resources and Services, a nonprofit counselling and information organization in Bala-Cynwyd, Pennsylvania, said women should also be warned about the profound consequences of hysterectomies before undergoing the operation. "The most frequent problems are loss of energy and stamina, loss of physical and sexual sensations, [and] diminished maternal feelings," she was quoted as saying. "It's very common to have urinary problems like leakage and increased urinary frequency. And the bowel moves down to take up the place where the uterus has been so over time it can become very difficult to have a bowel movement." However, guidelines by the Society of Obstetricians and Gynecologists of Canada say "there is no evidence in the literature that a hysterectomy leads to psychological distress. Sexual function is unchanged or improved in eighty per cent of patients following the operation."

Dr. Donna Stewart, director of the women's health program for Toronto Hospital, was on a task force studying the high rates of hysterectomies in Ontario. In areas where there are high rates of hysterectomies a fair number of these women are quite happy with the results, she said. "But do I advocate hysterectomies? No," said Stewart in an interview. "But there is a difference in values." Some of those differences in values are attributed to Catholic women. "It is a form of birth control for some women. And there are community norms. Once you finish your period, you get cleaned out, and some even say, 'I think I'll go to the clean-out doctor.'"

For others, it means saying goodbye to periods from hell, which feature unpredictable, heavy bleeding usually at the most inopportune time and not infrequently in a business suit. The problem is compounded when a woman lives in a rural or remote area. Although there are alternative treatments to hysterectomy, such as taking hormones, some don't like to fiddle with them—they're too busy working, caring for children and their parents, and so on. And the drive to a specialist can be a long one, especially in the winter when driving can be treacherous on ice-slicked, rural backroads.

Then there are women who have had a lot of children and whose uteruses have been stretched to large proportions. "There was once a woman who had a uterus this big," said Stewart in her office, using her hands to approximate the length of a small, oblong watermelon. "She'd had eighteen children." No argument there, for some women the uterus needs to be removed.

For these reasons, Stewart believes that hysterectomy rates should probably be higher in the north, but not two-and-a-half to three times greater than in Toronto. "I would try to encourage women to try hormones, to try more conservative methods of treatment," said Stewart, adding that the problem of heavy, unpredictable bleeding usually ends around menopause. Pain can be managed and prolapse can be fixed with a plastic ring inserted in the vagina and specific exercises. The bottom line, according to Vayda, is that "women living in Toronto have a much lower chance of getting their uterus out. No one can tell you this is all disease-related. It's largely a matter of treatment style; the path of least resistance."

After three years of study, researchers came to the same conclusion in a report entitled *Understanding the Variation in Hysterectomy Rates in Ontario*, which was released in February 1998. It found Ontario doctors were doing too many hysterectomies, partly because they are paid more money for surgeries than for using alternative methods to treat women with noncancerous uterine conditions. "The rate of financial reimbursement under [the Ontario Health Insurance Plan] makes it financially more rewarding to perform an abdominal or vaginal hysterectomy, which usually requires a relatively short period of time, compared to providing medical or alternative procedure care," said the report, a joint effort of Ontario's Ministry of Health and the Ontario Medical Association.

Unnecessary hysterectomies put women at risk and cost the health care system millions, but it is an inevitable outcome when a surgeon is paid substantially more to do a quick surgery, compared to spending months trying to perfect an alternative type of treatment, such as hormone medication. Dr. Fraser Fellows, co-chair of the task force that did the report, said he can sit in his office and listen to a patient's persistent complaints about heavy blood flow, problems with her sex life, and worries about the side-effects of medications for about $52, or "I can put a patient to sleep and take her uterus out in half an hour for about $250. The others are much more difficult to deal with than someone who is lying there asleep while I take out her uterus or fibroids."

In the U.S., hysterectomies are also very common: about 600,000 U.S. women have the surgery every year at a price tag of about $5 billion and at an average age of 42.7, according to Dr. Judith Reichman. Her book, entitled *I'm Too Young to Get Old: Health Care for Women After Forty* (Times Books), has placed the most common reasons for the surgery into one of four categories: necessary, acceptable, questionable (often not needed), and avoidable (definitely not needed). Her book urges women to fully research options and discuss their concerns with doctors.

The Ontario task force report had a similar finding, stating that women need to be given far more information on their condition and its alternative treatments, as they relied almost exclusively on the advice of their doctor. Few even knew there were other treatments for their ailments. "We need to bring people up to speed, not to be threatened or dictated to by their doctors," Fellows told the *Globe and Mail*. "They are not being told their choices, they are almost being dictated to."

A similar problem has been noted with Caesarean sections, a surgery that women usually have little control over. Although the Caesarean section rate in this country increased from about six per cent of deliveries in the early 1970s to almost one-fifth of deliveries in 1986, the rates dropped to about seventeen per cent in 1996. Although that's lower than the twenty-four per cent rate in the United States, it is much higher than the ten to thirteen per cent rate found in most Western European countries. The differences don't stop at countries: there are large differences between provinces, even though the mothers-to-be are not very different. For example, in 1991-92, almost one-quarter, or twenty-three per cent, of babies born in Newfoundland and British Columbia were delivered by Caesarean section, yet Manitoba and Alberta had Caesarean section rates of fourteen and sixteen per cent, respectively. "When used appropriately, a Caesarean section can be life-saving for both mother and baby," according to the Institute for Clinical Evaluative Sciences in Ontario's *Practice Atlas*. "However, if used inappropriately, this surgical procedure can put mother and child at risk."

The most common reasons for performing a C-section include having a previous C-section, slow labour, and fetal distress. Together, those three complications account for about three-quarters of all Caesarean sections. Although there has been a recent decrease in some provinces in Caesarean sections for women with slow labour or who have had a previous C-section, the rates for performing the surgeries for fetal distress have slightly increased over the past decade.

Dr. Stefan Grzybowski, director of research at the University of British Columbia, is working with several others to get the Caesarean section rate down in the province and in the B.C. Women's Hospital where he works in the family practice department. He has found that among the many things that can make a woman more likely to have a Caesarean section are "morbid fear of labour," a desire to deliver the baby on a "lucky day," pain, electronic fetal surveillance monitors on low-risk births, and admitting women to hospital too early in their labour. The hospital found that a good number of pregnant women admitted to hospital were not in active labour in that they were dilated less than three centimetres, said Dr. Susan Harris, medical program director of the low-risk birthing program at B.C. Women's Hospital. Thus, health care providers were under the impression that these women were in active labour longer than they really were. Consequently, doctors were more likely to perform a Caesarean section.

"I tell women, 'As soon as your contractions occur, I want you to write it down,'" Grzybowski said in an interview in Vancouver. "If you approach labour and birth as if everything bad is going to go off, then that's probably what's going to happen. Everybody is expecting the worst all the time."

According to Vayda, "The more elective the procedure, the greater the amount of variation." For example, it's clear when patients need operations to have their heart valves repaired and their brain tumours removed, but with operations that are more "elective"—such as hysterectomies and tonsillectomies—surgeons will vary widely on when the surgery needs to be done. So there's a much better chance of unnecessary hysterectomies and tonsil removals being done than there is of brain tumours being removed and heart valves being replaced. Vayda doesn't think these unnecessary operations are being done by "malevolent" doctors who are keen to cut. It's just that some doctors are more conservative than others, try drugs or other measures to treat the condition, and view surgery as a last resort; while others believe early on that the patient needs an operation. Vayda thinks "it's out of control with C-sections," as far too many of them are being done.

Guidelines that are followed by doctors are one way to ensure that surgeries are performed for sound reasons. In the late 1970s in Saskatchewan, practice guidelines for hysterectomies were developed, distributed, and combined with regular monitoring of doctors. These guidelines were developed at the urging of the provincial health minister after researchers pointed out a seventy-two per cent jump in the provincial rate of hysterectomies between 1964 and 1971, even though the number of women aged fifteen and older had increased by only eight per cent. A special committee of the College of Physicians and Surgeons of Saskatchewan was struck to establish criteria for when a hysterectomy was justified. They followed up their efforts by monitoring the medical and surgical practices in seven hospitals. As a result of those efforts, the province's hysterectomy rate went from one of the highest to one of the lowest, according to a study published in the *New England Journal of Medicine* more than two decades ago. In fact, the total number of hysterectomies in that province fell by one-third from 1970 to 1974.

Recent guidelines from the Saskatoon-based Health Services Utilization and Research Commission have called on doctors to stop giving asymtomatic men the prostate-specific antigen test for prostate cancer, since early detection has not been proven to lengthen lives. That resulted in a thirty per cent drop in the test. Unnecessary thyroid testing is also down in that province by thirty-five per cent. In 1997, the research commission released a report suggesting as many as twenty-five per cent of all chest X-rays, particularly those done routinely before a patient is admitted to hospital or before surgery, do nothing to help doctors or improve the health of patients, even though

250,000 are done every year. That kind of approach—aggressive monitoring and guidelines—could be tried in other provinces and would probably have good results, if there was the will to do it.

Guidelines on hysterectomies were released by the Society of Obstetricians and Gynecologists of Canada in 1996. The report noted that the outcomes most important to patients are "relief of symptoms, long-term complications, and effects on quality of life." When there is not enough evidence for doctors to agree on what treatment to follow for noncancerous uterine conditions, the "patient's preference is of major importance." Women in the northern and southwestern areas of Ontario are about three times more likely to have their uteruses removed, compared to Toronto women or those who live near medical schools. Hysterectomy rates are high in provinces such as Nova Scotia, New Brunswick, and Newfoundland, and lowest in Manitoba. Overall, Canada's hysterectomy rate is the second-highest in the developed world, just after the United States.

One area where doctors should follow clinical guidelines but don't is in treating and monitoring patients with high blood pressure. Yet estimates on Canadians with untreated high blood pressure range from 3.5 million to 4.1 million. High blood pressure is a risk factor for heart attacks, stroke, glaucoma, and kidney disease. Among those diagnosed, about forty-two per cent of cases are not being controlled, according to a study of 23,129 Canadians published in the *American Journal of Hypertension*.

"To be blunt, physicians haven't come up to speed on guidelines. We should be doing much better," study author Dr. Michel Joffres of the Department of Community Health at Dalhousie University in Halifax was quoted as saying in the *Globe and Mail.* "It is interesting that the lack of awareness of hypertension was generally not because people had not had their blood pressure measured, but was presumably because their doctors had not told them that the pressure was high," wrote Joffres. Medication and diet are key to controlling high blood pressure.

Joffres' study, which tracked patients with blood pressure from 1986 to 1992, found that only sixteen per cent of hypertensives were treated and controlled. A further twenty-three per cent were treated but not controlled, nineteen per cent were neither treated nor controlled, and forty-two per cent were unaware that their pressure was high. "It is particularly distressing that many Canadian physicians, despite knowing that their patients have hypertension, have elected to not treat patients adequately or, in some cases, not to even inform them of their hypertension," wrote Dr. Michael Weber, New-York based editor of the *American Journal of Hypertension.* So there are now two issues for patients: Not only are they uninformed about a potentially deadly condition, they are not being treated for it—one more reason to call high blood pressure the silent killer.

Another area where guidelines could help is Caesarean sections. In 1995, the Society of Obstetricians and Gynecologists of Canada released guidelines on the diagnosis and management of slow and difficult labour (dystocia) and fetal distress. The guidelines on slow labour stress the importance of correctly identifying when labour really begins and the need to monitor its progress. The group also pointed out how important it is for women in labour to have one-to-one nursing and other support as a way to reduce the need for a C-section.

That's particularly true when it comes to diagnosing fetal distress. Although it may sound like a smart idea to strap fetal monitors on every pregnant belly being wheeled through the revolving hospital doors, they can be easily misread or wrongly indicate that a fetus is in distress when in fact, it is not. Not only does the overall use of these monitors not result in better babies, it actually increases the Caesarean section rate. Still, they are routinely used in many hospitals in Canada. "Technologies applied routinely for two decades in North America, such as ultrasound and fetal monitoring, have not been shown to improve outcomes for low-risk births," wrote Sari Tudiver and Madelyn Hall in a paper entitled *Women and Health Service Delivery in Canada.*

The guidelines say that in most deliveries continuous fetal monitoring can be replaced by intermittent auscultation, the medical term for listening to the fetal heart at specific times during labour with a hand-held Doppler. Despite these guidelines, there is still wide variation on when doctors choose to perform Caesarean sections. "There are still many hospitals that have very high repeat Caesarean section rates even though the guidelines suggest that any hospital that provides routine obstetrical care should be able to perform VBAC [vaginal birth after Caesarean section]," said the *Practice Atlas*. In addition, hospitals seem to deal with fetal distress very differently—some opt for the Caesarean section right away, while others wait it out.

"The slow response of physicians to national guidelines has been observed in other contexts. Individual physician practices, hospital policy, type of hospitals, hospital resources, patient education, and patient demands could all influence the number of Caesareans that are performed," said a Statistics Canada paper entitled *Declining Cesarean Section Rates: A Continuing Trend?* "As well, concern about litigation may affect Caesarean rates. An increasing proportion of Canadian clinicians state that fear of litigation influences their decision to do Caesarean sections."

Dr. Gordon Guyatt, a Hamilton internist, had a study on guidelines published in the *Canadian Medical Association Journal* in 1997, with an eye to looking at who—if anyone—actually reads and follows them. He found most doctors don't, with only fourteen per cent of physicians surveyed saying they consulted guidelines on a daily or weekly basis, and less than a third saying they changed the way they treated patients as a result. That, even though there are currently about 2500 clinical guidelines in this country, and sixty-five per cent of the 1878 physicians surveyed said clinical guidelines are likely to improve patient care.

To be fair, there are many guidelines that sometimes contradict each other, which is off-putting to physicians. "I think there should be some kind of pressure on doctors to follow guidelines," Guyatt said. He concluded that "we need a consensus on what are guidelines backed by strong (medical) evidence … . Even so, one might have odd, exceptional situations where such guidelines might reasonably not be followed. Basically, where evidence is strong and values are uniform, I think there should be some kind of pressure on doctors to follow guidelines."

Most doctors don't follow guidelines, suggesting that the mere publishing of how to best treat patients is not good enough to make physicians change the way they practise medicine. Here again, the Americans do an excellent job of informing patients. There are many brochures available on medical trends and, in addition, one ingenious method.

The trustees of Dartmouth College set up the Foundation for Informed Decision-Making, which produces interactive video discs for patients to help them decide whether to get surgery or to follow more conservative medical treatment such as drugs or even watchful waiting, as in the case of an enlarged prostate. "Learning which [surgical] rate is right requires learning what informed patients want. The right rate must be the one that reflects the choices of patients who have been adequately informed and empowered to choose among the available options," wrote the Foundation.

The interactive videos, which typically run forty minutes or less, help patients make decisions on breast cancer treatment, prostate cancer, low back pain, and mild hypertension. They feature patients who have made decisions, and describe the harms and benefits of various treatment options. "It's not so much the choice of plan nor even the choice of doctor but the choice of treatment where the true empowerment of the patient begins," said Dr. John Wennberg, director of Dartmouth University's Center for the Evaluative Clinical Sciences in Hanover, New Hampshire.

One of the videos Wennberg and other researchers helped create was used on 713 Canadian patients with a benign enlarged prostate, as part of a University of Toronto and Toronto Hospital research project. The patients were at research sites in Victoria, Toronto, Winnipeg, Halifax, Vancouver, Oakville, Kingston, and two in Montreal. All of them had what is medically referred to as benign prostatic hyperplasia, a relatively common condition among older men. One of its symptoms is being awoken in the middle of the night with a need to urinate. Of the 664 patients, 31.5 per cent were classified as having mild symptoms, 47.6 per cent were in the moderate category, and 20.9 per cent had severe symptoms. Most, or eighty-three per cent, of the patients were fifty-five and older. And the group had a fairly high level of education: More than half had some post-secondary education, had completed university, or had an advanced degree.

There are various ways to treat a benign enlarged prostate, and it isn't clear whether surgery, medical therapy, or watchful waiting is best. Still, by 1989 surgery for a benign enlarged prostate was the second most common surgical procedure performed in North America on patients older than sixty-five. But surgery is not without its side-effects, which can include loss of sexual function and incontinence.

In Wennberg's interactive video disc, patients in the Canadian study punched in their condition, age, and a few other medical details and then heard the pros and cons of the various treatments, including viewpoints from patients who had received them. There was also a "learn more" section where patients could learn about how the surgeries are performed, various alternative treatments, the effects on sexual function, drug treatments, incontinence, among other topics.

Before seeing the video, 46.6 per cent of patients felt poorly informed about the risks and benefits of the various treatments. After the viewing, only 0.5 per cent still felt poorly informed, according to the final report of the BPH Shared Decision-Making Project written by Raisa Deber and Drs. John Trachtenberg and Allan Detsky.

Although many patients liked the video disc, they, unlike the U.S. patients, didn't change their minds about their treatments. Of the sixty patients who were leaning towards surgery before viewing the video discs, fifty-four still preferred it in the post-viewing questionnaire. Similarly, 356 of 401 patients continued to learn towards nonsurgical alternatives. Only 69 of the 203 remained unsure. "Our surgery rates didn't go down, but many people felt much better about their decision," said Deber in an interview.

Specifically, "we find that viewing the material has an effect on patient choice in less than one-third of the respondents to date. Not surprisingly, the effect is most pronounced for those who were initially undecided," wrote Deber and the other researchers. "This data suggests that strong preferences are less likely to change, although the intensity may vary, and that any changes which do occur appear more likely to move to 'undecided' rather than switch altogether. It was notable that of this preliminary group of patients, few who were strongly determined to have surgery or to have nonsurgical therapy changed their view as a result of viewing the program."

The most intriguing result for the researchers was how the relationship between doctors and patients improved. About six out of ten patients (58.5 per cent) said they trusted their doctor more after seeing the video. "Indeed, there was an even more positive response for patients … with 69.4 per cent agreeing that the video increases overall patients' trust in their urologist," researchers wrote. In conclusion, researchers found that "informed patients appear to be more satisfied. Genuinely shared decision-making need not threaten the doctor-patient relationship. It can enhance it." This interesting conclusion shows that information provided to patients not only helps them, it actually enhances their relationship with their doctors.

As patients, be mindful that, depending on where you live, there may be too many uterus, tonsil, and cataract operations being performed, to name a few. Find out if you are living in a surgical hotspot and include that information as just one more piece of the puzzle when making your decision on whether to go under the scalpel.

That said, it shouldn't exclusively be the public's responsibility to know if they are living in an area that does too many—or too few—of a given operation. Well-thought-out guidelines, drawn up by doctors and specialists in the field, should be followed with few exceptions. Guidelines and the doctors who do and don't use them should be monitored by committees of the College of Physicians and Surgeons in each province or a government-funded group of experts. That way, there would be not only a process to implement and track the guidelines, but the colleges could discipline doctors who refused to follow them without a good reason.

Patients, too, should be made aware by their doctors of other ways to treat ailments rather than surgery, which like any treatment, carries risks. All these things would make operating rooms a less busy place, or alternatively, free up time for surgeons to do operations that are much more medically warranted. But this is just one problem that occurs when doctors aren't monitored or tracked on their surgeries.

## QUESTIONS TO ASK

*Here are some questions to ask your doctor or surgeon. Remember: By the time you've made it to the surgeon, chances are you have already been deemed a patient who is likely to get an operation. You may want to ask these questions before you are referred for surgery. In many cases, guidelines on when to do various surgeries are on the Internet. Make an effort to find them.*

- What are the alternative treatments to surgery? What are the risks and benefits?
- What problems can I develop if I decline surgery?
- What problems can I develop if I choose surgery?
- Are there published guidelines about the treatment for my condition? If so, do you plan to follow them?
- Is the rate of surgery for this operation in this county or region higher than the provincial average? If so, why is that?
- What kind of anesthetic is usually used? Do I have a choice of anesthetic? What are the risks of being under an anesthetic?
- Will you be the doctor performing the entire operation? If not, who will it be and how much experience does he or she have?
- What kind of pain or discomfort will I be in after the surgery? How long will it last?

- Will I need to take medication after the operation? If so, what are the side effects?

## THINGS YOU CAN DO TO HELP

- Demand governments publish consumer guides pointing out the differences in surgeries by area and highlighting where they think there is too much or too little of it.
- Lobby hospitals and physicians to explore these differences and do something about them.
- Pressure government, hospitals, and the College of Physicians and Surgeons to encourage doctors to follow clinical guidelines.

*Eight*

# Cancer: Improving the Odds with the One in Three Disease

If you were to develop cancer, especially breast cancer, British Columbia is probably the best place to get it in. As devastating as a diagnosis of cancer is, what is also worrying is that the death rates for the disease vary from one province to the next. And that's not just for breast cancer, it's for colon cancer, prostate cancer, and many other types of malignancy.

"There's a remarkable variation between the provinces in what has been touted as a universal health care system but in fact is not," said Dr. Bill Hryniuk, former director of the Hamilton Regional Cancer Centre. Now a professor at the University of California in San Diego, Hryniuk said while some provinces are at the cutting edge of treatment for cancer, others are "way, way, way, way behind where they should be. These are differences the provincial cancer agencies would not like to talk about."

Some of those big differences have been observed in British Columbia, which in 1995-96 had a death rate for breast cancer that was thirteen per cent lower than the national average. For prostate cancer, it's six per cent lower and for colorectal cancer, it's thirty per cent lower. They ascribe their success to treating patients consistently according to what they know medically works. "Overall, this province has the lowest cancer mortality rate for males and the second-lowest mortality rate for females," according to their 1995-96 annual report.

For B.C., this is a very good news story, but it doesn't explain why patients there are faring so much better than in the rest of the country. Some researchers will bemoan the fact that more research needs to be done. They suggest that perhaps patients in the west coast are "healthier" or have better lifestyles and that having one of the oldest screening programs for breast cancer in Canada must have something to do with it. Another difference, however, is that the B.C. Cancer Agency has a policy manual, the *Cancer Treatment Policies Manual,* the only one of its kind in Canada. The manual is essentially an oncologist's user's guide on the latest and most effective treatments of cancer, and the majority of B.C. doctors are using it. As a result, patients across the province are receiving more consistent treatment. It is this consistent treatment that the B.C. Cancer Agency said was partly responsible for B.C.'s lower death rates for breast cancer patients.

"If you have breast cancer, this is a good province to have it in," said Susan Harris, a breast cancer survivor and a professor of rehabilitation sciences at the University of British Columbia. In 1994, a mammography revealed a tumour in Harris's breast that turned out to be cancer. She had a lumpectomy, what is commonly referred to as breast-conserving surgery, followed by radiation treatment, which helps cut down the risk of the cancer invading a second time. Because of the tumor's small size, Harris did not have to take any anticancer drug therapy, a decision that greatly affected her quality of life. "As a researcher, I respect the B.C. Cancer Agency guidelines because they are based on evidence," said Harris.

For his part, Dr. Don Carlow, B.C. Cancer Agency president, said he believes the *Manual* plays a role in reduced death rates. "Worldwide evidence suggests that the consistent application of treatment leads to lower mortality rates in cancer," said Carlow in an interview in his Vancouver office. "If you committedly apply evidence-based methods, you are going to have lower death rates."

The higher survival rates also have something to do with B.C.'s "broad-based cancer control mandate. Our cancer care is better developed in British Columbia than in other provinces. Before, everybody did their own thing. I guess you could say we're now a bit like McDonald's," he said. Although Carlow's analogy may sound like a bit of a joke, think about the suggestion for a moment: No matter where you go, the food at any McDonald's from St. John's, Newfoundland, to Surrey, British Columbia, tastes exactly the same, yet the treatment of cancer is not as uniform.

With a budget of $140 million, the B.C. Cancer Agency provides care through fourteen regional chemotherapy clinics and one provincial program in radiation therapy, so that the standards are as consistent as possible from one city to the next. As well, they believe their higher survival rates for breast cancer can be attributed to a three-pronged approach: self-examination, annual examination by a physician, and screening mammography. The B.C. Cancer Agency has mobile units to reach rural areas of the province (containing 3.7 million people) with what is called the Mobile Mammography Centre. But the province's good results aren't exclusive to breast cancer. Overall, B.C. has the lowest cancer death rate for men and the second-lowest death rate for women. If B.C.'s cancer mortality rate mirrored the Canadian average, there would be some 782 more deaths in 1998, the B.C. Cancer Agency projected. Of those, 102 deaths would be from breast cancer and 80 would be from prostate cancer. The total is the equivalent of two jumbo jets crashing and killing all their passengers.

And B.C. has the science to back up their claims. When National Cancer Institute of Canada researchers looked deeper into the data to find out why B.C. women had lower death rates than those in the rest of the country, they found that females at a higher risk of cancer recurrence in that province were more likely to receive anticancer drug therapy and those at low risk were less likely to receive it, compared to Ontario women. Specifically, eighty-two per cent of women under age fifty in B.C. at high risk of recurrence received anticancer drugs as recommended in the *Manual.* By comparison, only forty-two per cent of Ontario women in this group received the treatment. A study published in the *British Journal of Cancer* also revealed that eighty-five per cent of B.C. women under fifty at low risk of recurrence did not receive anticancer drugs, compared to seventy per cent who did not in Ontario.

What does that mean for women with breast cancer? "More women consistently receive good care here," said Dr. Ivo Olivotto, a B.C. Cancer Agency radiation oncologist, who co-authored the study with Drs. Carol Sawka and Vivek Goel of the Toronto-Sunnybrook Regional Cancer Centre and the University of Toronto. Olivotto is quick to point out that B.C. still has more work to do. "In B.C., across all ages, eighty per cent received chemotherapy and seventy per cent received tamoxifen when the guidelines recommended these treatments. We want one hundred per cent of patients to receive recommended treatments," said Olivotto, adding that "some patients aren't being referred to an oncologist and there are delays in the adoption of current guidelines in the communities." Olivotto believes the answer lies in awareness and education. "If we educate general practitioners, surgeons, and patients to be aware of provincial recommendations, we will further improve the consistency of care."

Even though there are treatment policies spelling out

to doctors the best way to treat cancer patients, doctors are not forced or even compelled to follow them. Carlow believes that forcing doctors to comply with treatment policies is eventually going to have to happen—it will just take time. He thinks the stick that will get doctors to follow the guidelines may be in funding: If oncologists don't follow the treatments as recommended, they won't receive remuneration.

Despite B.C.'s success, however, less than half of all women in the province between fifty and seventy-nine who should get mammograms actually do get them. "Imagine the impact we could have if we could increase the number to seventy per cent," said Barbara Kaminsky, chief operating officer of the Canadian Cancer Society's B.C. and Yukon division. Current recommendations for mammography suggest that women over the age of fifty receive a mammogram every two years to check for abnormal growths that may be early signs of breast cancer.

Shortly after the 1997 study was released, the B.C. Cancer Agency decided to beef up its efforts to track more women with breast cancer. Around the same time, it reviewed the Screening Mammography Program and found that it should be more active to recall previous women who had been screened, increase recruitment of women so that seventy per cent of the target population is screened, improve access to the service, and provide better information about screening mammography for women aged forty to forty-nine.

These differences in breast cancer survival rates are

something activists would like to know more about. Although the overall death rate per 100,000 females in Canada dropped to 28.4 from 31.9 between 1986 and 1995, some provinces fare dramatically better than others. British Columbia had the lowest rate with the death rate per 100,000 females at 24.2; Saskatchewan trailed in second with 26.1. Those two provinces did remarkably well, having the most striking decline in death rates of 3.1 and 3.4 per cent, respectively. "Things are improving but not at a rate most women would like," Kaminsky was quoted as saying in the *Globe and Mail.* Breast cancer death rates were highest in Nova Scotia (33), Ontario (30), and Quebec (28.9) out of every 100,000 adult females during the same time period, according to Statistics Canada's quality health reports, released in July 1997.

Dr. Barbara Whylie, director of medical affairs at the Canadian Cancer Society, noted that some provinces lag in areas such as mammography screening, but a federal program to promote screening should address that. In a news article, she was reported as saying the overall decline in breast cancer death rates is something to be happy about, noting that "it's been a consistent trend that's been maintained over at least ten or eleven years. It's significant." Whylie said the drop means that "we can win this war, but it will be won through a number of small incremental victories."

Despite the victories in Canada, Hryniuk, who left Hamilton for a post at the University of California, said that when it comes to breast cancer death rates, Canada "leaves something to be desired." There is a big difference in the breast cancer death rates among provinces, especially for women in the fifty to sixty-nine age group. "Thus, in this age group, mortality has declined by twenty-one per cent in B.C. [even better than in California] but has only declined by two or three per cent in the Maritimes and Ontario, and has increased by three per cent in Alberta. Manitoba, Saskatchewan, and Quebec show intermediate decreases of fifteen to sixteen per cent," said Hryniuk during the first Canada-U.S. Breast Cancer Advocacy Conference, held in Orillia, Ontario, in November 1996.

Hryniuk doesn't believe the differences in these death rates from one province to the next are due to underreporting of the disease or even to differences in virulence or incidence of cancer. "Although minor contribution may come from demographic differences, the most likely explanation for the variation may be that, in the past twenty years while advances in systemic adjuvant therapy [treatment following surgery] were being developed and introduced into clinical practice, these advances were unevenly applied to the women with breast cancer in the various provinces." As well, Hryniuk said the screening may not have been as consistently or rapidly adopted in all of the provinces as it might have been.

B.C.'s experience strongly suggests that when treatment policy manuals are developed and doctors follow them, patients get the best, most consistent care and live longer because of it. It's something that Ontario is also starting, with its implementation of evidence-based guidelines. This means that guidelines for treatments proven to medically work the most effectively will be distributed to doctors under the Cancer Care Program in Ontario. Although physicians do not necessarily have to follow them, the thinking is that they will, particularly since it is their peers—cancer specialists—who are creating them. A reduction in the death rates and better survival rates are two of the Cancer Care Program's objectives.

The Canadian Medical Association, in cooperation with Health Canada, has produced national guidelines for treating women with breast cancer in what some have called revolutionary fashion. Released in 1998, the guidelines come in two versions: One for doctors and a booklet for patients that is well-written and easy to understand. "This is nothing short of revolutionary," said Barbara Kaminsky, of the Canadian Cancer Society. "A critical issue for women is to be sure they have access to consistent, high-quality care no matter where they live." Health Canada has also formed a National Steering Committee to develop and implement the guidelines.

One can't help wondering, though, if publishing death rates not just by province but by health board or hospital would give patients more specific information that would compel them to shop elsewhere. The National Health Service in Scotland, for example, publishes one- and five-year survival rates of cancer of the trachea, bronchus, and lung; large bowel; and female breast and ovary by health board, leaving no mystery as to whose patients are doing best. The Scotland health service figures do come with this disclaimer, though: "It is stressed that no direct inferences about quality of care should be drawn from these indicators. They are intended rather to highlight issues which may require further investigation."

But probing the world of cancer care is never easy, especially for patients, some of whom are already feeling let down by the system. Worried they weren't diagnosed quickly enough or treated promptly enough, they feel their lives have been compromised. One woman who was in a high-risk group was so disturbed by how late her breast lump had been diagnosed, she was considering getting a prophylactic mastectomy on the other breast. "I feel let down by the medical profession because I don't feel my breast cancer was detected early enough. Women with a poor cancer history should be part of a select or different system of detection because of the high incidence of breast cancer as well as the fear of it," said the woman in a survey of breast cancer survivors for The National Forum on Breast Cancer, which took place several years ago. Another spoke of the despair at having to lobby for radiation treatment, which was to have begun early one October but was postponed due to long waiting lists. "I had to harass officials until I got my treatment, which started in mid-November. You shouldn't have to do this in order to get treatment! The anxiety is enough."

Cancer is a disease that conjures up images of something "growing inside" a person. "With cancer, it's a disease of the self," said Pat Kelly of Breast Cancer Advocacy Canada, a nonprofit organization, in an interview in

Burlington, Ontario. Kelly is a prominent figure in the cancer survival movement. Although she laughingly calls herself the "patient from hell," she is a person remarkably resilient and understanding, who is at the zenith of breast cancer activism. Despite her horrendously busy schedule, which includes raising two children and commuting to Toronto's Osgoode Hall to work towards a law degree, she also runs a Burlington-based office called PISCES, the acronym for Partnering in Self-Help Community Education and Support. There, she puts together a newsletter for breast cancer survivors.

She was also a key figure when survivors were asked to participate for the first time with scientists and doctors at the fall 1993 National Forum on Breast Cancer. She and other breast cancer survivors went to that landmark forum, armed with their own studies of those living with and surviving the disease. About 1150 women across Canada had filled out a questionnaire sent out by the Support, Networking and Advocacy Subcommittee, which represented women and their families with breast cancer at the forum. Interestingly, the responses showed that sixty per cent of women found their own breast lumps, either through routine examination or by chance. One-fifth, or twenty per cent, of lumps were picked up by mammography and an additional nine per cent were detected by the physician. Ninety per cent of women sought medical help within three months of noticing a change in their breasts. Sixty-five per cent were then diagnosed within one month and a further twenty-one per cent within three months. The National

Forum on Breast Cancer ended on a positive note: survivors not only felt they were being heard but had invaluable information about how they cope with the disease that scientists couldn't ignore. The final report of the forum recommended that a national network of support and advocacy groups be developed.

In addition to knowing basic things, such as the best treatment method, there are some questions cancer patients may not have thought to ask. For example, one would assume that the surgeons charged with the enormous responsibility of excising cancer would be doing lots and lots of the complex operations, particularly those physicians working in large urban centres. But that isn't necessarily so.

If one believes that practice makes perfect, a patient may not be keen to go to a hospital that does a very small number of cancer operations, particularly since half of all cancers are surgically removed. However, a 1997 study done by Dr. Neill Iscoe, a Toronto medical oncologist, shows that a large number of hospitals in Ontario are doing small numbers of high-risk cancer surgeries. Specifically, Iscoe found nineteen hospitals—both teaching and community—performed only one operation each for pancreatic cancer, even though studies have suggested patients fare better when high-risk operations are performed in centres that do a good number of the surgeries. And there's no reason why these operations shouldn't be done in centres that do more of them better, as the vast majority of cancer operations are not emergencies. Knowing their chances of survival are much better at another hospital, patients may opt to take the short trip.

Studies done in the United States have found that high volumes of high-risk cancer surgeries can make the difference between living and dying. A study published in the *American Journal of Medical Quality* in 1996 found that higher-volume regional hospitals in New York achieved "superior clinical outcomes to those at lower-volume hospitals" when performing the pancreaticoduodenectomy or Whipple procedure, which involves the removal of the pancreas. The Whipple procedure is a complex, high-risk operation performed largely on patients with diagnosed pancreatic cancer. Specifically, regional hospitals (tertiary care centres in New York) had an in-hospital death rate of 2.2 per cent, compared to 115 other community hospitals with a combined 12 per cent death rate, according to the study of 579 Medicare patients. That means patients who have the operation at a teaching hospital as opposed to a community hospital have their risk of dying cut a dramatic fivefold.

Dr. Pascal James Imperato, the study's author, noted that "this is probably due not only to the special technical expertise of operating surgeons at regional hospitals, but also to the availability and experience of nursing and house staffs and ancillary personnel. In addition, regional hospitals are more likely to have dedicated post-operative units with specialty support services capable of early intervention when complications arise."

With this study in mind, many patients could be

justifiably concerned about the low numbers of high-risk, complex operations performed in a hospital, particularly when it comes to cancer, where cutting out all of the malignancy is of crucial importance.

Despite its importance, Iscoe's study garnered only scant media attention. There was no press conference, and the 254-page scientific document filled with charts, references, and 1994-95 data was sent to few reporters. Still, it is full of interesting nuggets. A foreword written by Graham Scott and Dr. Leslie Levin says the study "underlines potential weaknesses in current practice by identifying areas where access may not necessarily be matched with excellence." While the pair patted some hospitals on the back for having major cancer programs, they also found that "low volumes of certain procedures are performed in some hospitals." This is particularly important in surgeries that are high-risk. "Everything we have learned about volume-outcome relationships in health care suggests that some complex procedures are best provided in centres where the surgeons have substantial experience, and where appropriately skilled teams are available to care for the patient."

One way to judge a surgeon's skill is to look at the volume of procedures a surgeon or hospital performs. While this won't tell you how good or bad a doctor or hospital team is, it does suggest whether a given doctor is performing enough operations to keep her or his skills up. As Iscoe points out, "high volume is rarely associated with poor outcomes." He also notes that "it has been suggested by some that the volume of surgery contributes to the maintenance of the skills of those involved in the care of patients." While chemotherapy, radiation, and support services are very important to cancer care, it should be noted that about half of cancers require surgery by a general surgeon or by a surgical oncologist.

The initial cancer study did not name the hospitals performing less than five a year of the higher-risk surgeries of the pancreas, liver, and lung, but it did name hospitals that performed less than five of three other types of cancer surgery. "The observation that there were DHCs [district health councils] in which the vast majority of cases were done at one institution with rare cases being done elsewhere is of concern. Does this represent the best care for these patients?" Iscoe asked.

He also pointed out that for "most cancer sites examined, there were a significant number of low-caseload institutions where cancer surgery was performed ranging from low-risk procedures [for example, bilateral orchidectomy for prostate cancer] to high-risk procedures [for example, pancreatectomy or hepatectomy]. Many of these institutions did not meet the eligibility criterion of five procedures in 1994-95 irrespective of a link to cancer."

"It would seem ethically and morally sensible to expect that patients be informed of alternatives that may result in different outcomes or levels of care and of the risks and benefits of these choices. The issue of outcomes [how well a treatment works], which has not been addressed in this monograph, is critical in making any determinations about the best locale for surgery," wrote Iscoe and co-authors Teresa To, Elaine H. Gort, and Michelle Tran.

To put it more bluntly, Dr. Charles Hollenberg, president of the Ontario Cancer Treatment and Research Foundation, told the *Globe and Mail,* that "there is absolutely no doubt in complex surgery that practice makes perfect. If any relative of mine had pancreatic cancer, I would insist they only have the surgery at a hospital that did a reasonable number of the procedures, even if that meant having my wife or my son or myself have surgery some miles away from home."

When it comes to prostatectomies, an operation to remove prostate cancer, Ontario hospitals within kilometres of each other varied in the number of surgeries performed, with eleven hospitals—all of them community hospitals—each performing less than five of these operations a year, according to Iscoe's research. A similar problem was noted with rectal cancer, as thirty-four hospitals did less than five of the operations a year. Unlike the previous example, mostly community hospitals did the highest number of these surgeries.

With rare exceptions, patients with head and neck cancers have surgery in teaching hospitals, a smart move considering it is difficult surgery that requires specialized rehabilitation afterwards. Even though ninety per cent of cases of cancers of the lip, tongue, throat, and larynx, among others, are referred to teaching hospitals, three Toronto community hospitals collectively operated on nine patients.

Iscoe speculates that patients may choose to have their operation in a particular hospital for personal reasons. That may have to do with the fact that it's nearby, that they or another family member has been in it before, or because they are very confident about the surgeon. Sometimes, a patient chooses a hospital that's very near to family—something of great importance that cannot be underestimated. "Knowingly or unknowingly, these patients may decide to have surgery in a low-volume institution," writes Iscoe. Most likely, patients aren't aware of how often a procedure is performed at a hospital compared to other hospitals in or out of their immediate area. But would that knowledge affect their choices?

Hospitals cannot always answer patients' questions about the number of surgeries performed by surgeon. "At present, very few hospitals or surgeons would be able to answer these questions, as the necessary data have not been readily available," writes Iscoe. "Should this information be part of the disclosure process prior to any elective procedure so that a patient can make a more informed choice?" Should it be the responsibility of the patient to ask these questions, or should it be the responsibility of the profession or the cancer care system to provide this information if it is available?"

While one could argue there is an onus on patients to ask questions, many more would suggest the onus should be squarely placed on hospitals. Not only should hospitals provide that type of information, but they should consider closing down low-volume programs. Although the overall quality of the health care system is very good, it "does not shed bad doctors, it doesn't get rid of low-volume and unsafe programs," said Michael Decter, former deputy minister of health in Ontario.

While the general public is intelligent, it is difficult as a patient to understand exactly what questions to ask. Most patients wouldn't think to ask how many operations a surgeon performs each year. They assume the hospital ensures that it's an appropriate amount to get good results.

For his part, Hryniuk believes that Canada's cancer system would be better if it was forced to publish five-year survival rates by cancer type and by hospital. The differences in death rates "may be partly due to unequal access," he said in an interview. But he is less in favour of controls that would ensure surgeons perform a minimum number of cancer operations to stay current. "I am basically not in favour of government regulation. Just publish their records and let the public decide."

When Hryniuk was asked what advice he would give to prospective cancer patients about their treatment, he said: "Get a second opinion from an American oncologist in a large cancer centre specializing in that disease." However, that may not be feasible for most Canadians, as it would be costly. Instead, try to find the top expert in your province. Hryniuk also stated that cancer patients should be sure to ask about *all* treatment options "regardless of whether or not they are applied in Canada." And don't be afraid to research your disease on the Internet, particularly on the home page of the U.S. National Cancer Institute.

To prevent "the continuation of uneven application of life-saving breast cancer treatment," Hryniuk recommended that "an immediate inventory be taken of the Canadian provincial care systems. A report should be generated showing what percentage of breast cancer patients at present have access to or are receiving screening mammography, adjuvant anthracycline-containing chemotherapy, tamoxifen, cytokines [G-CSF, GM-CSF], antiemetics, new drugs such as Taxol, and dose-intensive chemotherapy with stem cell rescue. Furthermore, open channels should be established for patients to access investigative treatments such as biologicals, pre-operative chemotherapy, and dietary studies."

Hryniuk said there are a few ways Canada could go. It could move to a completely private system; it could establish a national cancer control agency; it could force provincial cancer agencies to report outcomes directly to provincial legislatures in a public forum; and it could create a national volunteer coalition to continuously lobby the provincial and federal governments for improvements in outcomes. Of all the suggestions, Hryniuk believes the last two are most likely to be accepted and to work in Canada.

For her part, Kelly believes patients shouldn't be allowed to merely contribute to health care reform, but should be full voting members of all federally funded research granting agencies and cancer treatment centre boards of directors. That means having access to and information about the most appropriate diagnostic, treatment, and supportive care options, regardless of where they live in Canada.

As Kelly writes in her popular booklet, *What You Need to Know about Breast Cancer,* published by the members of the Burlington Breast Cancer Support Services: "You are the most important person on your cancer-care team. You are the one who must design your own treatment plan based on what you learn about your disease and from talking to others."

Although some still feel the need to study the effect of guidelines and policy manuals, there is enough evidence to suggest they help doctors provide the latest, most consistent treatment to patients. That's likely the reason British Columbia is doing better than the rest of the country when it comes to their patients successfully battling several types of cancer. More residents there are alive because of it.

Still, there are big differences in how well patients survive cancer that can be tracked by hospital and by province. Since patients aren't made aware of the differences in survival rates, they can't protect themselves. A report card would certainly help. Just imagine if these report cards contained information on the one- and five-year survival rates of patients. Patients could vote with their feet by not going to hospitals that didn't make the grade. And treatment guidelines would be enforced, not just encouraged.

## QUESTIONS TO ASK IF YOU HAVE BEEN DIAGNOSED WITH CANCER

- What type of cancer do I have? What stage is it at?
- Are there guidelines for the treatment for this type of cancer?
- What treatments are available? Where are they available?
- What is the prognosis if I take these treatments?
- What is the prognosis if I do not take the treatments?
- What are the side-effects of treatment?

*About half of patients who have cancer will undergo surgery. If you and your doctor decide you need an operation, you should ask the following:*

- Should I be getting this surgery at a teaching centre or at a community hospital?
- Is it better to have a surgical oncologist or general surgeon perform this operation?
- Is this type of surgery performed often? If not, how can I find a surgeon who has done a lot of them?
- Is there a surgeon who is specifically known for doing this kind of surgery well?
- If so, can I be referred to him or her?

## THINGS YOU CAN DO TO HELP

- Demand that cancer agencies and hospitals compel doctors to follow evidence-based guidelines.
- Lobby for standards so doctors are not allowed to perform low-volume, high-risk operations unless they disclose those facts to patients as part of informed consent.
- Push for the creation of cancer report cards so patients can see how provincial cancer agencies fare.

*Nine*

# When Being Treated Like a Man Can Hurt

Women are prescribed more mood-altering drugs, receive fewer kidney transplants, and suffer more fatigue than men. Women are afflicted with as many heart attacks as their male counterparts, yet they are referred far less often for open-heart surgery. Despite the popular cigarette slogan, women really haven't come a long way.

Often neglected in important studies because scientists fear their menstrual cycles will affect the results, women take drugs, receive operations, and are medically treated largely according to what is good for the seventy-kilogram, white male. That, even though they make up slightly more than half of the population and roughly seventy per cent of hospital visits. As Dr. Donna Stewart, director of the women's health program for Toronto Hospital, has pointed out, "Women are not just men with menstrual cycles. They are different; they metabolize drugs differently."

Specifically, an aspirin a day will help reduce men's risks of heart attacks and strokes, but no one knows for certain if this is true of women, as they were excluded from the large clinical trial, a type of research study that assesses the effectiveness of medical interventions. Similarly, women have largely been excluded from clinical trials of anti-ulcer drugs, sunscreen, anti-angina drugs, antibiotics, and anti-malaria pills. Even U.S. trials on Lupron, which is used frequently to suppress ovarian function, were conducted almost exclusively on men. And it's not as if this problem is new: Data taken from primate studies deal almost solely with the male baboon.

To do clinical drug trials almost exclusively on men is to make an inherent assumption that the male is the representative human being. That, coupled with paternalistic worries of fetal protection, has helped shut women out from being full participants. Oddly, the same protectionism hasn't been extended to men as subjects, even though taking part in drug trials could have an effect on their sperm. That said, the Medical Research Council has estimated about $34 million, or five per cent, of Canada's health research funding was spent on women's health issues in 1992-93. There were many limitations to the study, however, as the research council had difficulty obtaining all relevant data. Although funding records for 1994-95 don't reveal any major changes to the above figures, there at least appears to be a trend of funding more research with sex differences in the title.

To be fair, a similar study of research funding for men's issues estimated that only seven per cent of such monies goes into that sex's research, leading some to surmise that the remainder of research is neutral to both sexes and possibly equally beneficial to both. That would be an inaccurate assumption, given that men are able to benefit from studies when they represent the overwhelming number of research subjects in a way that women aren't. "Ignoring gender differences in the 1990s is somewhat akin to discussing lung cancer without reference to smoking, or claiming that aspirin protects against heart disease on the basis of data from a study of male physicians," wrote Patricia Kaufert in a paper entitled *Gender as a Determinant of Health.*

So fed up was David Dingwall, former federal health minister, at seeing only token women involved in clinical trials, that his ministry created a policy in 1996 that drug trials must be composed of men and women when a manufacturer expects to use the drug for both after it has been approved for market. Before the policy was created, Dingwall told reporters: "It can no longer be acceptable to have one hundred men in a clinical trial and have a token woman or two when they make up fifty-two per cent of the population. The era of tokenism has to end and end quickly."

Still, the worries of being a woman don't end at the clinical trial. There are many other areas where the health care system unwittingly discriminates against women, be it uneven access to care, too much intervention during childbirth, or improper prescribing during one's elderly years.

•

One of the areas in which women don't have equal access to health care is abortions. Whether these patients go to a teaching hospital or to a private clinic, they are likely to be harassed by pickets trying aggressively to dissuade them from getting the medical procedure, complete with brochures that show dismembered fetuses. And it's not just the patients who are harassed. So, too, are those providing the procedures.

In addition, there is another worry. Studies have shown that patients are more likely to suffer complications if they decide to go to a teaching hospital instead of a free-standing private clinic. In a 1996 *Canadian Medical Association Journal* study of women aged fifteen to forty-four who had 83,469 abortions from January 1992 to December 1993 in Ontario, author Lorraine Ferris wrote: "Compared with women who had an abortion in a free-standing clinic, the risk for immediate complications was greater among those who had an abortion in a hospital, especially a teaching hospital, a nonteaching hospital with 200 to 399 acute care beds, and a nonteaching hospital with fewer than 200 acute care beds."

With that in mind, the overall risk of immediate complications is still very low—1.3 per cent when a woman has the procedure at between nine and twelve weeks gestation, compared to 3.3 per cent for those who had an abortion at between seventeen and twenty weeks, according to Ferris's research. Put another way, an induced abortion is a safe procedure, but a woman is most likely to have the best results and lowest chances of complications in a private clinic.

"Unlike in previous studies, the woman's age, parity and history of previous spontaneous or induced abortions were not found to be risk factors," the study said. However, women who were advanced in their pregnancies or who had procedures that involved the infusion of saline (salt water) or prostaglandins, a substance that causes contractions of the womb, were more likely to experience complications, said Ferris.

While these findings can help guide those seeking an induced abortion, they work only for those who live somewhere abortion services are available. Even though Statistics Canada reports that abortions are the most frequently performed surgical procedure in this country, they are not easy for patients to get. The late Dr. Marion Powell, of Women's College Hospital, wrote in the *Canadian Medical Association Journal* in 1997 that there are thirty-two abortion clinics operating in eight provinces, but none in Saskatchewan and Prince Edward Island [1997 data]. In half of the provinces, women must pay out of pocket for the procedure. However, in British Columbia, Alberta, Ontario, and Quebec, abortion clinics receive full funding and the costs to women are covered under provincial insurance plans.

For women in need of an abortion in Prince Edward Island, it means taking a relatively long and costly trip to Halifax, Nova Scotia. As *Globe and Mail* health policy reporter Jane Coutts put it: "When you're faced with unwanted pregnancy, you're in for a trip: Abortion is not available in the province." Coutts travelled to P.E.I. and interviewed a number of women, including a thirty-two-year-old named Mary who already had two children and was pregnant with a third with her boyfriend. That was a surprise, given that she had been told that health problems had rendered her infertile. Mary, who did not want her real name used, could not afford another child and her relationship with her boyfriend was starting to fragment. "I am not a promiscuous person. I guard my health and my personal life in every way. And to get this medical care, I had to leave my home and drive for six hours," she was quoted as saying. The cost of the ferry, the hotel, medication, and gas was $400—all of which her boyfriend paid.

To be eligible for provincial funding in P.E.I., a woman must be referred to an out-of-province hospital, as no free-standing abortion clinics are funded by that province. The pregnant woman must pay the initial cost and then ask a board of three doctors to approve reimbursement—once again placing the medical establishment in the driver's seat when it comes to a woman's body. "Who needs it?" asked a woman named Liz in Coutts's article. "Asking a bunch of doctors to make decisions about my life ... I didn't even keep my bill."

Mary and Liz are fairly typical of those seeking abortions, according to a Statistics Canada report, although both were a little older than the average age of twenty-six. Only one in five women having an abortion is under twenty. Statistics Canada also found that sixty-nine per cent of women in their twenties who had abortions were single, as were one-third of women in their thirties.

Abortion is legal in Canada, but here's the kicker: When the law against abortion was struck down by the Supreme Court of Canada in 1988, P.E.I.'s legislature voted that any woman seeking an abortion must have the medical procedure in a hospital in addition to getting approval from a three-doctor board. According to the *Globe and Mail* article, in practice that means only five women a year—mostly those whose fetuses can be shown to have severe genetic defects—receive funding from the P.E.I. government. About two hundred women a year, many of whom couldn't afford to have another child, leave that province at their own expense in search of an abortion.

Even though these women do not have equal access, it is not seen as a breach of the Canada Health Act, as there is no requirement that every medically necessary service be offered everywhere. Although the province is within the letter of the law, one could easily question the compassion and politics of those who make it so difficult for women in need to get an abortion.

But this isn't just a problem in P.E.I. In Metropolitan Toronto, St. Michael's Hospital moved in April 1998 to quickly halt all abortions and vasectomies and restrict other birth control procedures at the former Wellesley Hospital site, which was ordered closed by the Health Services Restructuring Commission in Ontario. Long-time critics of the final takeover of the Wellesley Hospital were alarmed that one fewer facility in Toronto will be offering abortions.

"This is a very real concern and it's not simply a concern of just Wellesley, but speaks to other situations around the province," Carolyn Egan of the Ontario Coalition of Abortion Clinics told the *Toronto Star*'s Rita Daly. "Access has always been a problem and we haven't been opening up any more free-standing clinics."

Although most of Ontario's general hospitals have the capacity to offer abortion services, fewer than half do, according to a study published by the government-funded Institute for Clinical Evaluative Sciences in Ontario, which tracks the use of health care services in that province. While ninety-four per cent of Metropolitan Toronto hospitals surveyed offer the surgical procedure, only thirty per cent of those in northeastern Ontario perform abortions. The study of 158 Ontario hospitals also found that individual doctor preferences were a major determinant of whether a hospital offered the procedure. Almost fifty-seven per cent said the personal choice among doctors was the number one reason for not providing abortions, with the potential for harassment a distant second at twenty per cent. Almost one in twelve, or eight per cent, of hospitals who do not offer abortion services said they were picketed by demonstrators within the previous two years, while almost half, or forty-five per cent, of hospitals that provided the procedure reported experiencing some form of harassment. More than half of those who were harassed were picketed outside the hospital (53.9 per cent) and almost one-fifth (18.4 per cent) of the staff members were picketed at their own homes, said a study published in the *Canadian Medical*

*Association Journal.* Some hospitals that provide abortions received hate mail (10.5 per cent), harassing phone calls (9.2 per cent), and bomb threats (1.3 per cent).

These tactics are obviously designed to persuade hospitals not to perform abortions, and therefore give less access to women who choose or medically require the procedures. In some cases, it seems to have worked. But it's not as if difficulties end for women in the health care system when one decides to have children.

For decades, there were interventions or "things" done to women in labour in the name of routine, medical necessity. The most natural act in the world had become, over the past few decades, filled with unnatural acts, such as shaving of pubic hair, giving of enemas, and the controversial use of electronic fetal monitoring for low-risk births. Women also weren't all keen to assume unnatural labour positions during birth, such as lying on their back with their feet in stirrups. It all seemed so forced. Also, there was the assumption that once a woman has had a Caesarean section she must have one for all future births, which has been proven to be incorrect. Technologies that were supposed to help ensure a healthy baby—such as ultrasound and electronic fetal monitoring—were found two decades later not to have improved the medical outcomes for low-risk births.

A 1993 study entitled *Survey of Routine Maternity Care and Practices in Canadian Hospitals,* published by the Canadian Institute for Child Health and Health Canada, found that sixteen per cent of hospitals that responded had a policy stipulating that all women in labour should have a partial or mini shave of their pubic area, with small hospitals more likely to have this policy than large ones. Almost two-thirds, or sixty-five per cent, of all responding hospitals routinely used initial electronic fetal monitoring for twenty minutes to a half hour on all women on admission in labor. That same survey also found that eleven per cent of 523 hospitals that responded to the survey had a policy stipulating that all women should receive an enema or suppository—something that was also more likely in smaller hospitals.

Perhaps the most disturbing statistic of all was that episiotomies—done to enlarge the vaginal opening, particularly when forceps are used—were performed on a whopping sixty-three per cent of women having their first child and forty-two per cent of women who have had previous children, an excessive rate. "For decades, women silently questioned the necessity of such procedures and tried to regain elements of dignity and control over childbirth. Those who actively resisted, including some nurses and doctors, encountered opposition from professional associations and hospitals," wrote Sari Tudiver in her paper *Women and Health Service Delivery in Canada.* "Slowly, in the face of consumer pressure and mounting evidence against the need for routine interventions, changes have occurred in procedures in hospital settings."

But even for those who are knowledgeable, the changes are too slow. Savvy health care consumer Donna Kline, director of public affairs for Sunnybrook Health Science Centre in North York, knew a lot about the medical system.

Because she worked in a hospital, when she became pregnant she asked around for names of doctors to deliver her baby. Some things were essential to her. "I wanted a woman. If I'm going to open my legs 7000 times, I'd rather it be in front of a woman doctor. I also wanted that female doctor to have had babies of her own," Kline said.

After asking doctors at the hospital and friends who had children, she made lots of telephone calls trying to find a doctor who would be there to deliver her baby on her due date of August 12, 1997—prime vacation time for physicians. She finally decided on a family doctor who delivered babies, but not before she peppered her with a few questions. Upfront and blunt, Kline asked these questions of the family doctor she had heard about through friends: How many deliveries do you do in a year? Are you connected with the University of Toronto? How do you feel about C-sections and episiotomies? The answers were: about 150; yes, I have an academic appointment; and I don't do them unless they're necessary. These answers were comforting to Kline, who "wanted to make sure she was up to speed and current."

But there were other concerns. Kline, like virtually all women, didn't want to be cut unless she absolutely had to, so she pushed the doctor a little bit more on her feelings on episiotomies. "I don't think episiotomies are necessary," Kline told the doctor. "She said: 'You're right, a lot are done unnecessarily.'" Immediately, Kline felt not only at ease but that she was a partner in her health care at the all-women practice. She did jokingly mention, though; "'If I get a C-section unnecessarily, I'll sue you for every penny.' I was laughing, she was laughing. Ultimately, for me, it was about the doctor."

Babies, as it turns out, come out when they feel like it, the due date notwithstanding. Two weeks after her expected birth date, Kline, then thirty-four, went into a Metropolitan Toronto hospital to get induced. They started the process at 9 a.m. on August 25, 1997, with an intravenous drip that was to help put her into labour. But after twenty-one hours, her cervix hadn't dilated enough and there were problems with the position of the baby's face.

Not long after, things got rolling. "This strange guy walks into the room, he tells me I need a C-section and five minutes later, he's cutting me open," said Kline. But not before she told him a thing or two. "I told him I wanted a bikini cut, small and low." She also asked the obstetrician how many Caesarean sections he'd done before, and he replied, "Tons."

Kline had a local anesthetic for the Caesarean section, but it unfortunately wore off around the time the doctors were suturing her bikini-cut Caesarean section. "I was in excruciating pain as they were pulling my bladder out. It was an awful, horrible experience. But I don't know what could have been done differently. The people were good enough, proficient enough. The whole experience was completely unnatural to me. At some point, it felt like it was out of control." At the end of it, Kline and her partner André Turcotte had a baby girl named Gabrielle, eight pounds fourteen ounces.

After the surgery, when she was still in the hospital, Kline started to ask questions but found "information is not forthcoming. I think they think you should be glad you had a healthy baby. I think I'm going to requisition my medical records and read them. I want to know why I was in so much pain and why the baby didn't come out."

Even someone as savvy as Kline, who knew people in medicine and asked all the right questions, still had a lingering feeling that she wasn't informed as well as she could have been, particularly after the fact. At the same time, she did all she could to ensure the best outcome for her baby. No matter how some may try, though, women still have little control over the birthing process. At some point, a woman has little choice but to relinquish her body to the experts.

Heart disease, although seen as a "man's disease," is another contentious area for women. Even though heart disease kills as many women as men, women are often not diagnosed, partly because their symptoms are often more vague than a man's and are written off as stress, getting old, or hysteria. "Men and women do present [symptoms] differently," said Jennifer Price, a clinical nurse specialist in cardiology at Women's College Hospital in Toronto. "Men, they have crushing chest pain. It goes down their arm and it usually occurs with exertion." Only forty per cent of women have those so-called typical symptoms known to men, while the other sixty per cent have symptoms of tightness, burning, and a little heaviness in addition to the more subtle signs of neck pain, back pain, and shortness of breath. Price points out that heart disease can often be missed in older women who go to doctors complaining of fatigue and not feeling so well. "They [patients] don't realize it themselves, sometimes. They think it's part of getting old," said Price.

There is also a feeling among women that heart disease is still very much a man's disease. Although many women believe the most common killer of their gender is breast cancer, it is actually heart disease. In fact, heart disease was the leading cause of death of Canadian women in 1996, killing 131.7 out of every 100,000. That compares to the breast cancer death rate of 28.6 per 100,000 females, according to Statistics Canada figures. The real risk for heart disease comes after menopause, because before that estrogen protects a women; after the so-called change of life, "there are problems with blood clotting and arteries don't respond as well," said Price.

Besides the worry of not being diagnosed early or properly, there is the problem of finding a surgeon who is good at operating on women, which isn't as easy as it sounds. In some surgical circles, there is a feeling that women are not great candidates for coronary artery bypass graft surgery because their hearts and vessels are smaller, which makes it more difficult to operate on them. Other surgeons don't like operating on women because they don't get as good results as they do with men.

Women who are diagnosed with heart disease at Women's College Hospital and need surgery will inevitably be referred to one of two surgeons at Toronto Hospital: Dr. Linda Mickleborough, Canada's first female cardiovascular surgeon, or Dr. Tirone David. While David is well known as probably one of the best heart surgeons in the world who does complex cases, particularly valve surgery, Mickleborough has superb results operating not only on men but on women. A study of 1132 men and 355 women who underwent bypass surgery found that only slightly more [1.4 per cent] women died compared to [1.1 per cent] men.

The study, published in the scientific journal *Circulation*, found that women were not necessarily more likely to die during surgery than men, even though female patients were older and were suffering from more illnesses, although Mickleborough and others did qualify the findings by noting that the women she had operated on had had less extensive heart disease than the men.

Despite those impressive results, several recent studies have found that women are less likely to be referred for the so-called "revascularization" procedures, which include coronary artery bypass graft surgery and angioplasty, a non-surgical procedure in which a catheter with a balloon tip is inserted into the artery to widen it. "Concern over increased operative mortality in women should not bias referral patterns for angiography or coronary bypass graft surgery," wrote Mickleborough in *Circulation*. "More studies are needed with large numbers of female patients to examine sex-specific risk factors for coronary bypass graft surgery."

Dr. Len Sternberg, chief of cardiology at Women's College Hospital, said women are less likely to receive angiography, a procedure in which dye is injected into the coronary arteries to detect blockages that might be treatable by surgery, but he isn't certain why that is. "It may be that women aren't getting equal treatment, or we may be overusing the procedures in men," said Sternberg.

After analysing the angiography test results of 575 patients, of which one-third were women, Sternberg found "more normal angiograms among the female patients, which suggests that heart disease in women may be different somehow or at least harder to diagnose non-invasively." However, once normal tests were excluded, "we found no significant difference in the number or severity of blocked coronary vessels. The fact is that women do develop serious heart disease."

In 1995, Dr. Susan Jaglal, assistant professor of preventive medicine and biostatistics at the University of Toronto, and her colleagues conducted a study of Ontario patients referred to a group practice of cardiologists. They found that forty-eight per cent of women had stress testing done by the referring doctor, compared to seventy per cent of men. "Numerous studies in Canada, the United States and Britain have consistently shown that women with CHD [coronary heart disease] are less likely to be referred for invasive diagnostic and therapeutic procedures as compared with men," Jaglal was quoted as saying in *The Medical Post*.

Another study of women referred for less invasive cardiac testing found that women were twice as likely to have their symptoms attributed to other causes by their family doctor, and were less likely to be referred to a cardiologist if they were labelled as having psychological problems.

Even when women are rushed to emergency after suffering a heart attack, they are not given the same drugs as men. A major advance in treating heart attacks is the immediate use of thrombolytic or "clot-busting" drugs such as tissue plasminogen activator (tpa) and streptokinase. But research suggests that even though women obtain the same benefits of reduced mortality and less heart damage as men on the drugs, they are less likely to receive thrombolytic drugs in the hospital emergency room.

One other problem is that while women may be good nurturers, they can be notoriously bad at looking after themselves, sometimes putting off the inevitable. In one case, Eleanor Cameron had a vague feeling of discomfort in her chest in January 1995 and promptly went to her family doctor. Well past menopause at age sixty-four, she was sent to a cardiologist, who did an angiogram and stress test before figuring out that she needed heart surgery. At the time, Cameron was busy in her job as an office manager and had too many other things to think about: a husband with newly diagnosed prostate cancer and grown children she didn't want to worry. In some ways, she couldn't fathom the idea that she had heart disease, particularly since she exercised every day during her lunch-time walks. How bad could it be? "I just didn't want to go. I thought I would put it off," she said afterwards. Cameron opted for medical therapy, thinking she could make do with a prescription for nitroglycerin tablets.

Not long after, she felt a vague discomfort in her chest during her daily, forty-five-minute lunch-time walks. Not pain, she insisted. It just felt different, uncomfortable somehow. Could it be her heart? Although she had been told to get her heart checked out before, the recommendation seemed more like a distant bell. She had put it in the back of her mind, filed away until she got everything else under control. But that distant bell was now an alarm.

She made an appointment with her family doctor who promptly referred her to a cardiologist, who did a stress test on her in January 1997, with the surprising result that "I couldn't do it. I was really sore," said Cameron, who also had an angiogram. "When I went back, they told me I had a plugged vessel. The doctor told me he was going to make an appointment with a surgeon." After hearing the news, Eleanor and her husband wept in each other's arms in the doctor's office.

The next stop was cardiac surgeon Dr. Linda Mickleborough, who told Cameron in her no-nonsense way that she needed triple bypass surgery. "I kept thinking, 'Why me?' but then I realized, 'Why not me?' I've been so lucky throughout my life. I was never sick before that. The only time I had been in the hospital was to have my two sons." Scheduled for surgery four months down the road, in May 1997, Cameron decided to take the extra time to make out her will and get herself psychologically clean by telling those she loved, particularly her sons Joel, thirty-two, and Terry, thirty-three, how much they meant to her.

So organized was Cameron that every week she drew

up a list of things that needed to be done: Get the VCR fixed, clean the cupboards, use up the gift certificates, clean the cobwebs from the basement, buy presents, fix the railing, make notes for appointments, and arrange home care if necessary. Each week, Cameron would check off one item at a time, sometimes revising her list before her big surgical date with Mickleborough. "I just wanted everything clean and neat."

The surgery was a success, and not long after Cameron started a rehabilitation program at Women's College Hospital, set up specifically to address the low rates of heart attack recovery by women. Ironically, as many as one-third of Canadians who have had a heart attack receive little or no follow-up care after they are discharged from hospital. And while women are referred to rehabilitation programs less often than men, they are twice as likely to drop out of them. "Our problem in Canada is the appalling gap between guidelines and practice. While patients get great care in hospital for the few days after the heart attack, what happens to the patient over the next two to three years? That's where we're falling down," Terence Kavanagh, medical director of the Toronto Rehabilitation Centre, was quoted as saying in the *Globe and Mail.*

Generally speaking, rehabilitation combines diet advice with a moderate exercise program, medication, and learning ways to reduce risk. Typically, recovering heart attack patients do ten minutes of warm-up, followed by twenty to thirty minutes of moderate aerobic exercise and then a cool-down, two or sometimes three times a week.

However, a survey of family doctors found only sixty per cent of them knew patients should be referred to exercise programs and only twenty per cent were aware of the current guidelines for medication, according to results of questionnaires given to general practice physicians by George Fodor of the Ottawa Heart Institute. That, even though another study showed that those who continue with an exercise program can reduce their risk of a second fatal attack by at least twenty per cent. "We're not berating doctors or giving them a report card," Kavanagh said. However, Fodor pointed out, "there are things that should be routine that are not."

Research done by Dr. Heather Arthur, associate professor of health sciences at McMaster University, found that while sixty per cent of men are recommended for rehabilitation by their physician, only about thirty to forty per cent of women are. "Then, the question is how many show up," said Arthur, at that time a research fellow at the Heart and Stroke Foundation of Ontario. Although fewer women attend the rehabilitation sessions, some say it's because they are designed largely for the convenience of men. "Often they are, and women cite family responsibilities or lack of transportation for why they don't attend," Arthur was quoted as saying in the *Globe and Mail.* Arthur also found that while half of men tend to stick with their rehabilitation program, only one-quarter of women do. "That's because they feel out of place. In one study I did, a woman told me she felt she was a 'curiosity' in a class of twenty men," Arthur told a reporter.

Unlike men, whose wives often accompany them to rehabilitation sessions, women have fewer support systems. "We don't see husbands showing up with their wives at cardiac rehab sessions," said Price in a leaflet called *Heart Disease Primer for Women,* distributed by Women's College Hospital. "Older women with heart disease are often widowed or alone, while younger women tend to put their family's needs ahead of their own." Some women also report receiving negative messages from their doctors about the benefits of rehabilitation, yet men are encouraged to enter rehabilitation programs, which teach them how to modify their risk factors for further heart disease.

It's something that virtually all heart attack patients could benefit from. Fodor estimated that at least a third of Canadian heart patients are not reaping the benefits of recent discoveries about heart attack recovery, he told reporters. The knowledge gap could be partly due to the fact that scientific evidence on drugs and rehabilitation is relatively new. In one example, the effectiveness of lipid-lowering drugs has only been known since 1994.

Instead of thinking they're lousy exercisers who won't participate in rehabilitation, Women's College Hospital created a program for women with heart disease with an eye to keeping them there. In a room the size of a small gym, women walk the treadmills, work the exercise bikes, and do exercises for their upper body. But all of them are working towards strengthening their bodies and minimizing their risk of a second attack, usually by attending two sessions a week for about six months.

"We do tailor-made programs for the women here," said Karen Unsworth, exercise coordinator of the Women's Cardiovascular Health Initiative at Women's College Hospital and a kinesiologist. "After rehabilitation, they will be able to increase their functional capacity by twenty-five to thirty per cent." This prediction is consistent with research that shows women seem to bounce back from bypass surgery as well as men do. Harvard Medical School researchers studied 436 female and male bypass surgery patients and found that women reported similar or greater improvements in daily living, mental health, and vitality to the men.

From the family doctor's office, to the cardiologist, to the actual heart surgery, and then to rehabilitation, women face biases at every single stage of dealing with the very serious condition of heart disease. It doesn't take a clinical trial to figure out that some doctors are not as up-to-date on how this disease affects women as they should be, nor do they seem keen to refer women to rehabilitation as often. That's why it's important for older women who are at risk of heart disease or young diabetic women who are also at increased risk, to be mindful of vague chest pains and not to write them off as part of the aging process, stress, or anxiety. Although a doctor may have the best of intentions, it doesn't necessarily mean he or she will provide the best care.

Biases in the health care system for women don't end with heart disease. As women get into their very senior years, they experience the problem of being overdrugged. As one gets older, the chances of being prescribed more drugs grows—particularly if one is a woman. In fact, elderly women are more likely than other groups to be prescribed sedatives and mood-altering drugs. It's such a problem that the Canadian Medical Association published a policy in 1993 that stated that "several studies have found that physicians' prescribing knowledge for elderly people is often inadequate and inappropriate prescribing is common."

Research studies suggest one in five hospital admissions can be attributed to an older person with a drug-related illness, with improper and overprescribing fingered as the main culprits. Although these hospital admissions were initially thought to be because elderly patients metabolize drugs differently—which they do—researchers now believe the main problem is that far too many prescriptions are being written for the aged. As the Canadian Medical Association's preamble to their policy pointed out: "In elderly people, adverse drug reactions are often complex and may be the direct cause of at least twenty per cent of hospital admissions for acute care."

Regardless of hospital admissions, studies vary on how much drug-prescribing is inappropriate. Some research suggests eighteen per cent of prescriptions for the elderly are improper, while others point to a high of fifty per cent. In particular, women are given more of the so-called psychotropic drugs, which include antidepressants and anti-anxiety medication, and benzodiazepines such as Valium and Librium.

One of the most comprehensive Canadian studies on

this phenomenon was done in Quebec, where researchers probed the prescriptions of more than 63,000 elderly patients, those aged sixty-five or older, in that province. With the exception of heart drugs, the "female patients were exposed to significantly more high-risk prescriptions than the male patients," wrote the researchers in the *Canadian Medical Association Journal* in a 1994 article. Specifically, elderly women were given more benzodiazepines (sedatives) and psychotropic drugs (mood-altering medication), while the "prevalence of high-risk prescribing was higher among the women than among the men and increased with age," said the study by Robyn Tamblyn and others.

In fact, more than half, or fifty-four per cent, of the Quebec women received at least one prescription for mood-altering drugs as compared to forty per cent of the men. Of those people, about three-quarters of the men and women also received the sedative-type drugs. So rampant was the prescribing of Valium-type drugs that a full one-third of elderly Quebec patients were on them for more than thirty days during the study period in 1990. "In summary, we found that high-risk prescribing was common in the elderly population and that questionable prescribing of psychotropic drugs was the most prevalent form of high-risk prescribing," researchers wrote. "We suspect that questionable high-risk prescribing may contribute to an increased risk of drug-related illness in elderly people," they said, adding that questionable prescribing for the elderly needs to be explored.

Despite other studies with similar findings, no one seems to know why doctors are overprescribing. However, there are big dangers associated with the practice: elderly people on drugs that make them drowsy can fall and fracture their hips, not to mention the potential problem of their becoming addicted to their medication. Also, since so many of the elderly are on medications, mixing them is not a good idea and can land them in the hospital with toxic combinations. Notwithstanding all this evidence, little is being done to change this improper prescribing.

There is one constant to this problem, however. No matter what age one is, the common denominator for receiving more mood-altering drugs and sedatives through life seems to be being a woman—it just gets worse as one grows older.

Once again, these are areas in which there is little to no accountability in the health care system. A system exists where women are receiving drugs they don't need for illnesses they don't have, yet they can't always get a proper diagnosis, medication, and testing for areas where they really need it, such as heart disease. Despite dozens of studies pointing out these types of serious problems that directly affect women's lives, little has been done to change or educate doctors about them. And patients, in this case women, are the ones paying the price for it.

## QUESTIONS FOR WOMEN TO ASK

*If you are having a baby, there are questions you need to ask about your care. The Society of Obstetricians and Gynecologists of Canada has developed guidelines for managing labour and delivery. Make sure you and your physician are aware of them.*

- If I had a Caesarean section before, do I need another one?
- How do I know if I'm in active labour?
- What can we do to make sure my labour doesn't last too long?
- Does your hospital supply one-to-one labour support? If not, why not?
- Are you going to use continuous electronic fetal monitoring? If so, why?
- In what circumstances should I expect an episiotomy?

*If you are being prescribed medication, ask:*

- Has this drug been tested on women?
- If not, how do I know it will work on me?
- Do I really need tranquillizers or mood-altering drugs? I hear that women have been given too many of them. (This is particularly important if one is an elderly woman.)

*If you have symptoms of heart disease, such as vague chest pains, shortness of breath, or unusual fatigue, tell your family doctor. Also ask him or her if you could have heart disease.*

*If referred to a cardiologist, ask:*

- Am I going to have a stress test? An angiogram? If not, why not?
- Am I being referred for cardiac surgery? If not, why not?

*If you are being referred for cardiac surgery, ask if you can be referred to a surgeon who is reputed to have good outcomes on women. This is extremely important. Be insistent.*

## THINGS YOU CAN DO TO HELP

- Lobby the federal government for equal access in all drug and surgical trials.
- Advocate for better access to cardiac services, be it diagnoses of heart disease or actual heart surgeries.
- Lobby governments to monitor the overdrugging of the elderly and to educate doctors about the hazards of it.

*Ten*

# Casualties of Cuts

There are two things a patient in need of medical care shouldn't be in Canada: old and poor. That's arguably the worst possible combination when seeking access to medicare. What's the best mix? Rich. Any type of rich will do. Elderly and rich, young and rich, middle-aged and rich. Just have money. For some reason, wealth seems to ensure access to hospitals during a time of massive downsizing in a way nothing else does. It's as if the affluent are on some golden Rolodex of hospital admissions that the rest of the ailing don't know exists.

As crude as this sounds, the methods to get on this golden list are not. It's not as if bribes are taking place, bank account balances are required upon admission, or operating rooms only accept platinum credit cards. It's far more subtle than that. Choices are being made on who gets care, and it is quietly eroding the foundation of a health care system that promises equal access to all. It's not supposed to be that way. Canadians are proud of their medicare legacy and its central tenet of treating all equally. And when times were good and provincial governments were providing double-digit increases to hospital budgets, that was mostly true. Now that times are tight, it's true no more.

A University of Toronto study by scientist Dr. Geoffrey Anderson that tracked downsizing in Ontario hospitals—the province in which some of the most dramatic hospital cuts have taken place, next to Alberta—suggests the poor are bearing the brunt of the cuts. While politicians and some scientists attached to government-funded bodies like to trot out flattering figures that more day surgery is being done than ever before—a statement that is categorically true—they neglect to mention just who is reaping the rewards of better access to care. Either they don't know, or they don't want the public to know.

That is one of the ironies of science. What figures may seem to show at first blush—that hospitals are doing more with less, and Canadians need not worry—looks very different when one goes deeper into the data. To analyze those figures by income group is to see the dark side of medicare: to see what happens, albeit unintentionally, when fiscal times are tight and there's only so much medical care to go around.

First, the big picture. Canada has lost more than 51,000 staffed beds (beds available for use by patients), going from 172,425 in 1986-87 to 120,774 in 1994-95, the latest figures available. That's the equivalent of closing 200 hospitals of 250 beds each. The greatest loss of beds was seen in acute-care hospitals where more than thirty thousand beds were cut over the same time period. On a population basis, that means 30 per cent or almost one-third fewer beds per one thousand people, according to *Downsizing Canada's Hospitals,* a Statistics Canada Health Report published in spring 1997.

In recent years, hospital spending across Canada has dropped about 2.5 per cent per year. Hospitals feeling the hit include those in the provinces of Alberta, New Brunswick, Ontario, Prince Edward Island, Quebec, and Nova Scotia. Exceptions are Saskatchewan, British Columbia, Manitoba, and Newfoundland, provinces that have seen increases to their budgets. British Columbia's growth is reflected in its population boom, which far surpassed that of any other province, according to the Statistics Canada report written by Patricia Tully. For the most part, provincial governments have finally achieved their goal of spending less on hospitals, and some are even looking at doling out a little more in future years.

Although the average length of a hospital stay in Canada has dropped from nine days in 1986-87 to seven days in 1994-95, the amount of outpatient care has predictably soared. The argument goes like this: Patients are staying in hospital for shorter periods of time than ever before. Although these patients are leaving hospitals earlier, they're just as sick—they're just ill at home, with or without follow-up home and nursing care. And many who would have stayed overnight are now able to leave on a so-called day basis, typically within twenty-four hours.

As drastic as cuts to hospital inpatient care have been, there have been huge increases in other areas. Day and night care—defined as care for outpatients, those on geriatric day care, those receiving renal dialysis, and substance abuse day or night programs—has jumped forty-six per cent; surgical day care has increased to thirty-seven per cent; the use of clinics has increased by twenty-four per cent; and emergency visits have crept up a tiny one per cent over a seven-year period, according to the same Statistics Canada report that tracked hospital use from 1986-87 to 1993-94. Downsizing would sound like a smashing success if the interpretation of statistics ended there. After all, Canadians are spending less and it appears they're receiving more. But that's only part of the story.

When Anderson examined how downsizing in Ontario affected people by income group, medicare started to lose its universal flavour. While those living in census divisions with the lowest incomes (the poor) in Ontario have always been admitted to hospital far more than those living in census divisions with the highest incomes (the rich), the gap is narrowing. (In explicit terms, the poor are described as those living in areas of Ontario with household incomes of an average of $38,800, or those in the lowest twenty per cent of household earnings. The so-called rich or wealthy are those living in areas where the average household income is more than double that at $78,800, or the top twenty per cent.)

Now, let's look at who is really feeling the pinch of downsizing. The moneyed have seen an eighteen per cent decrease in the rate of inpatient admissions to hospital medical beds and a twenty-three per cent drop in being admitted for surgeries that require more than a day's stay, from 1991-92 to 1996-97 in Ontario hospitals. It sounds like the rich are paying their fair share until one investigates what kind of decrease in hospital services the poor have taken. The lower income groups had a twenty-five per cent decrease in admissions to inpatient medical beds and a twenty-nine per cent decrease in admissions to inpatient surgical beds. Since these are percentages, one can say that the poor have been disproportionately affected compared to the rich. Put another way, both groups saw cuts in overnight stays in medical or surgical beds, but the poor experienced these cuts in a more dramatic way.

"The Canadian health care system has traditionally prided itself on removing financial barriers to care through its universal health insurance system," wrote Anderson in his paper published in *Medical Care*. "The analysis of hospital admittance revealed a gradient in hospital separation rates across income quintiles, with lower income groups having higher separation rates ... but the finding that the gradient across income groups decreased between 1991-92 and 1995-96 raises some questions about the changes in the equity of health care delivery in Ontario during that time period."

If that wasn't enough, the rich saw an increase of twenty-six per cent in day surgery, but those living in the poorest areas saw a three per cent *decrease* during the same time period, according to the research. So far, those in the lower income groups have been hit twice: once by a decrease in admissions in inpatient medical and surgical beds and then a second time with less access to day surgery beds. Yet, one assumes that these poorer people must still take ill—they're just not turning up in the health care system in the proportion they did before.

Let's take a look at a few procedures to see if there is some consistency to the hypothesis that the poor are getting less. When it comes to hip and knee replacement surgery—operations with some of the longest waits in the country—the Ontario poor did see an increase of thirteen per cent. Not bad until one notes that the rich experienced a hefty forty-one per cent increase for the surgery, which is typically done on the elderly.

It's the same when one looks at life-saving heart surgery. While the poor experienced a twenty-nine per cent increase in so-called revascularization procedures such as coronary artery bypass graft surgery and angioplasty, the wealthy saw a thirty-seven per cent increase. The same goes for cataract surgery: The poor saw a fifty-five per cent rise in it, while the moneyed class experienced an eighty per cent ascent. In other words, the most affluent members of society saw more than a threefold increase of hip and knee replacement surgery, a twenty-five per cent increase in heart surgery, and a fifty per cent increase in cataract surgery over their poorer counterparts.

Worse things can happen if one is not only poor but also old. If one analyzed the drop in care by age alone, one would find that the elderly with lower earnings had a seven per cent decrease in medical beds and a thirteen per cent decrease in inpatient surgeries. That compares to elderly wealthy patients who saw a one per cent decrease in the inpatient medical beds and an eight per cent decrease in inpatient surgeries. While old people—no matter how rich or poor—saw an increase in day surgeries, the wealthy experienced the lion's share of the increase in what is becoming a depressingly familiar statistic. Although the lower income people saw a twelve per cent increase in day surgeries, it was the elderly, wealthy groups that saw a twenty-one per cent increase during the time period of 1991-92 to 1993-94.

The long and short of it is this: It appears the poor are shouldering most of the cuts to the health care system. Scientists and the public know in general that poor people are far sicker than the moneyed classes because they frequently don't have good housing, nutritious food, or jobs where they are in control and make a reasonable salary. Consequently, the poor have always received more hospital care under medicare. But for how long? New figures show that the poor or those with less than half the average household income are getting far less hospital care than they used to, while the rich are getting just as much or more. So much for equal access no matter how rich or poor. Tommy Douglas would be appalled.

No one really knows why this is happening. Certainly, no one is consciously deciding that these patients are not worth treating. But could it be that doctors are more likely to do diagnostic tests on, recommend surgeries for, and admit those patients who are most like themselves? Perhaps, but it's hard to say. Or is it that wealthier people are more savvy with the medical system, thus demanding more investigations into their conditions, which means more surgeries and treatments? That's also difficult to know.

Anderson's study isn't the only one to look at the effects of hospital downsizing. In 1996, Noralou Roos, a co-director of the Manitoba Centre for Health Policy and Evaluation, and other researchers found that although the number of beds in Manitoba was cut by close to twenty per cent, more people were treated than ever before. Although Roos didn't find out whether people felt the care was good, she and other researchers found patients were no worse off because of the cuts.

"We carefully reviewed hospital use between 1989 and 1994. The first of the bed cuts took place in 1992," said Roos in an Atkinson Letter, published by the Atkinson Charitable Foundation. "In trying to determine if quality of care deteriorated, we had to identify indicators of trouble. We asked physicians and nurses what they worried about. They were concerned that patients discharged from hospital too soon in an unstable condition would suffer complications that would bring them back to the emergency room. But we didn't find that shorter lengths of stay in hospital led to more problems after patients went home."

How could two studies come up with such different findings? The answer likely lies in the depth of the cuts in Ontario, compared to those in Manitoba. Manitoba is tied with Saskatchewan for having the most acute-care beds with four per one thousand people in 1994-95, according to Statistics Canada figures. That's almost double the amount of acute-care or short-term beds Ontario had, with only 2.2 per one thousand people for the same time period. In fact, the only province with fewer acute-care beds than Ontario was British Columbia, which had 2.1 per one thousand people. So while Manitoba has felt cuts to the fat of its hospital system, the cuts have not been nearly as dramatic as those observed in Ontario, where it seems to many that they have gone down to the bone. It may be unfair to apply a Manitoba study where cuts were smaller, to Ontario where the cuts were extraordinarily deep.

However, Roos did have a note of caution on her study: "I think we have to keep monitoring to make sure we don't go too far. A study in the U.S. found that if you let the bed situation get too tight, those who are less able to negotiate the system—usually the poor and the middle class—will be less likely to get the care they need."

In its mildest form, the Ontario study suggests that the principles of medicare are not being applied, as the poor aren't getting the same care as the wealthy members of society. And there's no reason to believe that other provinces behave any differently towards the most vulnerable members of society. The only difference is that Ontario actually studied the issue.

Where you live and how much you earn are connected to whether you develop cancer. People who live in poorer areas are stricken with more lung cancer and cancer of the head and neck than those who live in richer areas. Still, the wealthy don't get off that easily—they develop more cancers of the brain and breast. But according to a study done by Dr. William Mackillop, a Kingston radiation oncologist, the chances of surviving cancer are always lower if you live in a poorer area.

Specifically, Ontario patients living in communities with median incomes of less than $20,000 annually were far less likely to have five-year survival rates in cancers of the breast, cervix, prostate, uterus, bladder, esophagus, head, and neck than those with household incomes between $30,000 to $40,000. But those in the $50,000-plus range had the best survival rates of all, according to the study published in the *Journal of Clinical Oncology* in April 1997. "While Canada's health care system was designed to provide equitable access to equivalent standards of care, it is clear that residents of rich and poor areas do not experience identical outcomes once they develop cancer," wrote Mackillop. "In poorer communities, there is both an excess of cancer deaths and an excess of deaths from other causes," said the study, which tracked 357,530 cases of invasive cancer diagnosed in Ontario between 1982 and 1991. "This should not occur in Ontario's publicly funded, single-tier health care system. However, we have shown differences in the management of breast cancer between rich and poor communities in Ontario so that possibility cannot be ruled out."

Mackillop was referring to a study of 46,687 female

breast cancer patients, that found those with a median household income of less than $20,000 were fifteen per cent less likely to receive radiation treatment within one year of being diagnosed with a tumour than those with an average household income of more than $50,000. Lead author on the paper Dr. Lawrence F. Paszat scrutinized female breast cancer cases diagnosed in Ontario between 1982 and 1991 and found that while "older women may have more severe comorbidity and/or different preferences for treatment compared to younger women ... the decline in RT [radiation treatment] utilization rates begins at age forty. The associations are consistent with observations about decreased BCS [breast conserving surgery] rates and decreased RT utilization for breast cancer in older women in the U.S." Paszat's study also found those aged fifty-one to seventy had a 16.9 per cent lower likelihood of receiving radiation treatment within one year of diagnosis. Those aged seventy-one and older had it the worst of all, as they had a sixty-six per cent lower likelihood of receiving radiation treatment within one year of diagnosis.

Quite simply, a disturbing pattern was developing: The older a patient got, the less likely she was to receive radiation treatment, commonly used after breast-conserving surgery as a means to kill any remaining malignant cells. That's surprising, since older patients with breast disease—particularly those fifty and older—should be more likely to get breast-conserving surgery and radiation treatment. After all, mammography screening for women that age and older has been proven to be more effective at detecting cancer.

Therefore, one would suspect a higher proportion of women over age fifty should be eligible for breast-conserving surgery plus radiation treatment. "Older women with breast cancer may be treated differently than younger women for reasons unrelated to the disease, and these reasons may include [the] relative barrier to their access to radiation treatment," wrote Paszat. Could it be that the elderly are also being discriminated against?

Mackillop's study found that there was a significant "excess of deaths" of many forms of cancer—not just breast cancer—in those who have lower so-called socioeconomic status, or who earn less than wealthier Ontarians who also have tumours. No one is certain why this is, but some speculate that the poor are more preoccupied with the scramble for everyday survival than they are with noticing minor changes in their bowel habits or blood that came up in a cough. Since so many cases of cancer begin subtly with night sweats, a cough, or fatigue, the poor may have trouble distinguishing them from a case of the flu or feeling run down from a lousy diet. According to Mackillop there are three possibilities: Poorer patients could have more advanced or serious cases of cancer once they are diagnosed; they could have other ailments that make surviving cancer more difficult; or "it is possible that residents of poorer communities may receive inferior care."

Of the three possibilities, Mackillop believes the least likely scenario is that the poor are being given inferior care. However, he said it is just as unsavoury if poor people are being diagnosed late or not going to the family doctor until the symptoms of cancer are more obvious. "The usefulness in this [study] is that it might allow you to target needy populations," said Mackillop, who has testified on Canada's health care system to the U.S. Ways and Means committee.

Mackillop speculates there may be "differences in the way the well-to-do are handled" as opposed to the way poor people are handled, once they reach the family doctor's office. "Well-to-do push harder and general practitioners may respond in a different way. There's a sense that you're actually in control of your life. Richer people enjoy a greater degree of empowerment," he said. If a doctor sloughs off a patients' worries of feeling unwell, the "rich are more likely to push and say, 'I really don't feel well,'" he said in an interview.

Conversely, with poorer Canadians, there's a scramble for survival. If a slovenly patient who reeks of body odour comes in complaining of poor bowel habits, would a physician automatically think "cancer"? Or would that same physician be more likely to think "cancer" for a three-piece suited businessman who has taken time out of his "busy schedule" to make a special doctor's appointment to complain of blood in his stool? Although the bias may not reveal an inherently poor character flaw, it doesn't matter how ill-intentioned the move may or may not be, as the outcome is the same: less care for the poor. Which is the exact reason why Mackillop did the study—so the less fortunate can be targeted for treatment.

Other studies suggest that people respond best to those in their same "socioeconomic group," a delicate way of saying those who come from the same social and income class. Poorer people are seventy per cent more likely to get lung cancer than their wealthier counterparts, yet it is the poor who are less likely to survive the disease five years later. Specifically, thirty-six per cent more of the richer people with lung cancer were alive five years later compared to the poor, according to Mackillop's study.

Head and neck cancers, including those in the lips, tongue, oral cavity, gums, salivary glands, tonsils, and throat, are more prevalent in poorer populations, yet richer folks with household incomes of $50,000 and up had a thirty-eight per cent better survival rate than the group with median household incomes of $20,000 or less. That means more than one-third of richer folks were surviving the rapid-growing cancer five years later, compared to the poorest group.

Patients with cervical cancer in the highest-earning groups also had a twenty-five per cent better five-year survival rate than those with $20,000 or less household incomes. The same goes for prostate cancer. And breast cancer patients in the highest income category had a nineteen per cent better five-year survival rate than those in the lowest income group. Those living in communities with $50,000-plus household incomes had a twenty-five per cent better survival rate of cervical cancer; a twenty-three per cent better survival rate for uterus cancer; a twenty-seven per cent better survival rate for bladder cancer; and a whopping 117 per cent better survival rate for esophagus cancer compared to those in the lowest household income group. Interestingly, the use of radiation varied widely from one region of Ontario to another. Its use ranged from a low of 24.5 per cent to a high of 44.4 per cent.

Since the cancers weren't itemized by their stage (the cancer registry doesn't track stages yet), Mackillop can't say with absolute certainty why richer Ontario patients are waging the war against cancer with more ammunition than their poorer counterparts. One thing is indisputable: Although wealthier Ontarians survived cancer far better than the others, "in none of the fifteen disease groups were there any signs of a trend in favour of the residents of poorer communities," said Mackillop. "Universal medicare doesn't overcome the difference in health between rich and poor. There's more to health than illness care," he pointed out, referring to previous studies that show poorer women are less likely to get pap smears than wealthier ones.

The poor and the old aren't the only ones discriminated against. Unlike those two groups, others do make it past the hospital doors only to be quickly whisked out of them again. This is especially common if one is a woman who has just given birth.

With increasing frequency, moms and their bundles of joy are being sent home from hospitals within twenty-four hours of having an uncomplicated vaginal delivery. Though this practice works well if there are backup home services available for the mom and tots, there aren't always, leading some to dub this trend as "drive-through deliveries." Even moms with complicated births are being sent home within twenty-four hours, when they really should be staying in hospital for longer than that. That was certainly the case for Irene Santos. Giving birth was supposed to be one of the most beautiful experiences of her life, filled with wonder and awe. She had counted on it being painful, even a little frightening, as this was her first baby. But rushed? A little more than twenty hours after a difficult forceps delivery and an episiotomy that required fifteen stitches, Santos was sent home from a Metropolitan Toronto community hospital with daughter Kayla Alexandra Benjamin on September 26, 1997.

Santos's husband Henry Benjamin was on a special project at work and couldn't get away. Her parents have busy careers and had a difficult time getting any time off until the second week, when her mother was able to help out. This wasn't exactly the entry into motherhood the thirty-year-old had dreamed about. It was hectic, confusing, uncertain. "It's not what they teach you in labour preparation classes," said Santos. "The preparation ends at the point you go into the hospital. It doesn't touch on anything after the fact."

Once at home, the pain was so great, Santos said: "It felt like I was never going to walk again in my life. It was horrible." Although a public health nurse did provide two visits—more than many other mothers receive—it wasn't nearly enough. Santos subsequently hired a private nurse from St. Elizabeth Health Care to come into her home for one week from 9 a.m. to 1 p.m. "I had to get a treatment because I had developed an infection. I think they should have let me stay in the hospital for one week. It was a bad time. I couldn't have done it alone. I just wonder what happens to mothers who don't have the money to pay a nurse," said Santos, who paid $15 an hour out of her own pocket for the nurse, while private insurance picked up the rest. "Having a baby isn't like getting your tonsils out. To have a baby and take care of yourself within a day is too much." Her advice to mothers: "If you can afford it, get help for the first week or two because you're going to need it."

The Society of Obstetricians and Gynecologists of Canada has recommended women who have had a "complicated labour and vaginal delivery" stay in hospital three or more days if there are no home care services available. If those services are available, staying in hospital at least two days or more is recommended. "There have been numerous reports, including three randomized controlled trials which have shown early discharge [within twelve to forty-eight hours] with appropriate follow-up in the home results in a low and acceptable rate of readmission of mothers and babies," according to the guidelines produced by Dr. Nan Schuurmans. "The experience in the United States with very short length of stay with no follow-up has shown poor outcomes with unacceptable rates of admission [fifteen per cent] for mothers and babies."

When sent home too early, some babies have to be readmitted to hospital with jaundice and dehydration, with its tell-tale signs of a sleepy baby who has little appetite. Dehydration is usually caused by insufficient feeding and is not uncommon in women who are sent home early, as their milk can take a week to start flowing. If not treated, dehydration can cause brain swelling and brain damage. A study of seventeen-year-old boys has suggested that moderate levels of jaundice are associated with decreased intelligence.

A study by a Hospital for Sick Children researcher published in the U.S.-based *Journal of Pediatrics* found that between 1987 and 1994, the number of infants readmitted to Ontario hospitals after being stricken with dehydration and jaundice during the first week of life more than doubled. In two cases, the babies died. Specifically, the study found the readmission rate for babies during the first seven days of life in 1994 was 13.2 per 1000 live births—more than double the 6.5 per 1000 rate in 1987, according to researcher Dr. Kyong-Soon Lee, a neonatologist. Hospital readmission rates for infants also increased substantially during the second week of life, from 6.4 per 1000 newborns in 1987 to 7.5 per 1000 in 1994. "Babies were coming in very sick with dehydration and jaundice," Lee says of her experience at Sick Kids. "There were a couple of catastrophes where infants died of dehydration." The study also found a "greater severity of jaundice in the infants readmitted to [Sick Kids] during the seven-year period."

The biggest study ever undertaken in the U.S. on early discharge of mothers and their newborns found, perhaps quite predictably, that they had a much higher chance of being readmitted to hospital within the first month of life than those who stayed longer after delivery. The *Journal of the American Medical Association* study, published in July 1997, followed more than 310,000 infants discharged within thirty hours of birth from U.S. hospitals. "Given these findings, we estimate that among healthy newborns at least eight of every one hundred rehospitalizations within the first week of life may be attributable to early discharge or may be preventable if the risk of early discharge was eliminated," Dr. Lenna L. Liu and colleagues wrote. Those at increased risk for having to go back to hospital following a thirty-hour or less discharge included first-born infants; mothers younger than age eighteen; and mothers with premature rupture of membranes.

Widespread concern that this practice of sending mothers and their babies home within twenty-four hours has compromised safety has led to national legislation in the United States, mandating coverage of a minimum forty-eight-hour hospital stay. In Canada, there is no such legislation, but some are taking the money saved from reducing the length of hospital stay following birth and putting it back into home nursing care.

By 1994, when many this country's hospitals were sending more and more moms home early, North York General was one that did more than pocket its $600,000 a year in savings. The hospital, which delivers more than four thousand babies a year, decided to fund a program at $300,000 annually to provide follow-up care in the home. North York General nurse Susan Kwolek, who runs that program, said hospitals have gone from one extreme of keeping mothers in hospital for a week to sending them home too quickly. "This is a natural body process. Women want to be more in control. Doctors aren't gods any more.

But the pendulum has swung too far the other way," said Kwolek. "To get a public health nurse, it varies depending on where you live. Some mothers have to be at risk to get a follow-up visit, while others don't." Consequently, some doctors deem mothers to be at risk when they're not, just so they could get the follow-up visits of a public health nurse for their patients. In the North York General Hospital program, moms and their newborns who are discharged within twenty-four hours are seen by St. Elizabeth Health Care nurses for two follow-up visits in the home and they are entitled as many phone calls to these nurses as they like for one week.

By fall 1997, the program had been going a full year and while the readmission rates to hospital for newborns had not dropped significantly, only two mothers had returned to hospital for care. In that year, the hospital had seen twenty-two babies readmitted for jaundice, eight for medical complaints, and eight more with dehydration. But, as Kwolek pointed out, the readmission rates could have been much higher had they not started the program.

As hospitals close by the dozen, programs are being merged and nurses are laid off by the thousands. At last count, there were 978 hospitals across the country in 1994-95, according to the latest Statistics Canada figures available. That's 246 fewer hospitals than in 1986-87. But the figure changes almost monthly.

Will I be able to get care when I need it? Am I being sent home too early? Who is going to pick up the slack?

Those are just a few questions many are wondering as they try to figure out what these hospital closings will mean when they take ill.

Deep cuts in Alberta mean public health spending has plummeted to the lowest level in Canada, with the provincial government spending only $1588 per person in 1997. That's $150 less than the national average and $367 lower than the top spender of British Columbia, according to figures from the Canadian Institute for Health Information, an independent, nonprofit body set up to provide comprehensive health figures. Before the cuts, in 1992, Alberta spent $1924 per head, the highest level in Canada and $107 more than the national average.

Alberta New Democrat leader Pam Barrett said she found the figures "staggering and painfully sad," according to the *Edmonton Journal.* But Alberta Health spokesperson Garth Norris wasn't surprised by the figures, adding that Alberta was the "first to take clear and firm action to get its spending under control. Now that's finished, the province is already reinvesting in the health care system, while many others are only now getting spending under control," Norris was quoted as saying in the *Journal.*

The Alberta branch of the Consumers Association of Canada also had its own report on that province's health care cuts. The consumers group found that people were taking time off work to spend it with relatives and friends who, while hospitalized, had trouble getting even basic needs met, such as help going to the washroom and getting a call button answered. In its 1996 report entitled *Taking*

*Stock: A report on the risks to consumers (and their employers) from current health system reform in Alberta,* the group found "some felt that they were expected to carry too much of the load for medical care in the hospital and at home, especially when they weren't really confident they were doing the right things. Long waits for certain tests or surgeries, and difficulties getting specialist medical care were all mentioned. So was the stress level of staff."

In large part, the lack of care in all hospitals across Canada reflects the thousands of nursing jobs that have been cut. "What we're seeing is a decrease in the quality of care. The burden is being passed on to families," said Mary Ellen Jeans, executive director of the Canadian Nurses Association, adding that this is what happens when cuts to the health care system are "fiscally driven."

Certainly, a crisis of public confidence in the medicare system was taking place, not just in Alberta but elsewhere. This was confirmed when a government-appointed watchdog body, the Provincial Health Council of Alberta, found that health care reform has left nearly half of its citizens dubious about whether the system will be able to care for them when they get sick. As well, Albertans were spending more of their own income on health-related care than they did five years ago, including costs for eye examinations and health-insurance premiums. Specifically, the 1997 report said the average Albertan spent $663 during the 1996-97 budget year compared with $596 in 1992-93, an increase of eleven per cent (based on 1992 dollars). Albertans also had trouble transferring between hospitals in the province and weren't sure where they should get treatment for mental health problems, according to the report of the council, which was appointed in 1995 to give advice to government on its health care restructuring program.

In what has been considered the biggest single health care upheaval in Canadian history, in 1997 Metropolitan Toronto was slated to close eleven out of forty-four hospitals in a process that is supposed to take several years. News of the closings has been marked by protests, court challenges, and threats that patients won't be able to get necessary medical care when all of the hospitals close. Of all the protests, the loudest have been heard at Women's College Hospital, which was initially against merging with Sunnybrook Health Science Centre but has since worked out an agreement. By the year 2000, Metropolitan Toronto residents will get care in new megahospitals, specializing in treating the sickest of the sick. As well, there will be specialized services to care for those in the home.

Although there is no equivalent watchdog of hospital restructuring to that in Alberta, other groups have attempted to track the effects of downsizing, including the Ontario Nurses Association, a union that did its own questionnaire of 277 patients. Although the Nurses Association stresses that the 1997 questionnaire is not scientific, it noted a litany of complaints from people who said "care is starting to fragment all over the place," said Lesley Bell, chief executive officer of the Ontario Nurses Association. "The most vulnerable are definitely not getting the care that they used to. When an 86-year-old has to start taking care of her 102-year-old mother who had a hip replacement, you know there's something wrong."

Even the little things one would take for granted, such as basic toiletries, aren't always there. One woman was told to pack a pillow, toilet paper, and facial tissue before her major cancer surgery at a Metropolitan Toronto teaching hospital —evidence to her that times were tight. Not only have patients been told to bring in their own toilet paper for years, but now they're also being told to bring in their own towels. "There are no clean towels to be washed with. Of course, that's if anybody even offers to wash you," said Bell.

In response to the nurses' questionnaire, patients complained that they had difficulty getting the care they needed, that the quality of health care they had received had declined, and that few professional care providers were available to deliver front-line care at their community hospital, nursing home, or community health service agency. Four out of ten respondents said they have had to look after or pay for the care of an acutely-ill relative at home. One Ingersoll, Ontario parent was upset that her daughter had to sit at home on a holiday weekend from Friday to Tuesday with a badly fractured ankle in a splint, as there was no one available to operate on it. Another in St. Catharines was disturbed that her father, dying of cancer, was in a hospital that had "few nursing staff; little clean linen; no basins readily available to catch bodily waste." The stories went on and on.

Today, according to Bell, the hope is that "there is someone at home to catch patients sent home early," and some physicians are even advising relatives of patients to hire a private-duty nurse because the nurses left working in hospitals are being spread too thin, she said. "The acuity [sickness] is so high in patients in hospitals now. There's just not enough nurses any more."

That certainly seemed to be the case for Robert MacLean, a widower living in Etobicoke who developed a hernia. Shortly after he came home from hospital in late fall of 1997, he fell and blacked out. Although it took some time and two more hospital visits to figure out what had happened, it turned out that when eighty-three-year-old MacLean fell, he had ruptured the operation to repair his hernia, which caused internal bleeding. Eventually MacLean was sent home and his daughter-in-law Jill made arrangements to have a private nurse care for him. Later, a variety of home care services would be purchased, including a cleaning lady and a nurse's aide. For an eight-week period, the bill came to a whopping $8000.

Ethel Meade, chair of the health care issues committee for the Toronto-based Older Women's Network, said she knew of a woman in her seventies who was instructed before her scheduled hysterectomy to show up at the hospital with her private parts "already shaved"—something she and her husband had to figure out for themselves. "Can you imagine that? Would you even know what to do? This is a woman in my generation," said Meade. Among seniors, the word is "don't go to hospital alone," she said. And if a patient does? "People won't see you. You will lie there and wait. You have to have someone be your advocate."

Another big centre closing hospitals is Montreal, which began this process in earnest in 1996. A year later, it had closed seven hospitals in a restructuring plan that involves cutting $190 million from that city's twenty-eight hospitals. Once complete, the new hospital system will have 2438 fewer beds, will have transformed two hospitals into long-term care facilities, and will have amalgamated six hospitals into two giant medical centres linked to universities.

From Victoria, B.C., to St. John's, Newfoundland, almost every hospital is changing the way it serves patients by treating more of the ailing on an outpatient day basis. Some hospitals have even benefited from the changes by becoming bigger and absorbing smaller institutions or their programs. Although these changes aren't bad in themselves, this period of upheaval has undoubtedly left some with less care.

As hospitals have been cut, much of the focus has been on the combination of a megahospital that treats the sickest of the sick and the need for home care services. Spending on home care has exploded, growing at a rate of about twenty per cent per year in the last two decades in Canada, according to Health Canada's *National Health Expenditures in Canada* (1975-94). The dramatic growth in spending in home care is triple the inflation rate, and by 1998, home care costs are expected to reach $3 billion in Canada.

Although home care is seen as the wave of the health care future, Dr. Peter Coyte of the University of Toronto warns that the evidence that it works isn't in yet. "A disturbing aspect of the growth in home care spending has been the lack of compelling evidence that home care services are a cost-effective alternative for institutional care," wrote Coyte in a study he did on home care in Ontario. "While a recent review of the international literature concluded that the provision of home care was associated with a small to moderate reduction in the need for, or use of, hospital days, other studies have shown this relationship to be weak."

Shortly after those comments, the Saskatoon-based Health Services Utilization and Research Commission released the first Canadian study comparing patients convalescing in hospital to those who rest at home following medical treatment. The study of 780 Saskatchewan patients found that patients recovered just as well at home as they did in hospital, at far less cost. "By continuing to use hospitals as the site of choice for convalescence, we aren't allowing home care to do its intended job," Stewart McMillan, chair of the commission, said of the study released in March 1998. "Our findings suggest we're using hospitals as a costly substitute for home care."

Despite that positive study from Saskatoon, there's another problem: Not all patients get the same access to home care. At least that's the case in Ontario. Coyte's study found that the use or availability of home care varies greatly across Ontario. The lowest rates are in Metropolitan Toronto and the nearby regions of Peel, Durham, and York. He and other researchers looked at how many patients received home care within thirty days of being discharged from hospitals from 1993 to 1995. Home care was defined by researchers as comprising at least one visit by a health professional within a month of leaving hospital. The statistics, which were adjusted for age and gender, showed as much as a thirty-threefold difference in the rate of home care available to patients, depending on where they lived.

Overall, only four per cent of same-day surgery patients were sent home with home care, compared to thirteen per cent of in-patients, but when it was broken down by area, huge discrepancies were found, said Coyte of the study prepared by the Institute of Clinical Evaluative Sciences in Ontario, a government-funded body that tracks the use of health care services in that province. For example, in the musculoskeletal category, which includes rehabilitation from orthopedic operations such as hip and knee replacements, forty-two of one hundred patients in Kingston received home care, compared to Metropolitan Toronto, which had roughly fifteen out of one hundred. There were many other comparisons of those who received home care after cataract surgery, a hysterectomy, or having their tonsils removed. The discrepancy can be partly explained by whether the physician orders home care and by whether home care is even available in the community. When home care isn't available, the burden predictably falls on families, particularly on women.

Many of the complaints about the health care system come from those who have stayed in a hospital and received treatment. However, one can't help but wonder about those who never get as far as the local hospital. The poor, the elderly, and the destitute appear to be the main casualties of deep hospital cuts, with those groups seemingly not getting the same access to heart surgery, cancer treatment, or knee replacements as their wealthier counterparts.

Although no one knows why these people are not getting the same care, the reason doesn't much matter. It shouldn't be happening; patients should be targeted to get the treatment they need and deserve. And it isn't hard to find them: They are the have nots in society, living in the poorest areas, in the worst conditions, eating the most unhealthy diets, without the benefit of a higher education. Others are elderly men and women living on pensions, trying to get through their twilight years as frugally as possible.

It is peculiar that a health care system built almost exclusively for these people is now not serving all of them. Unwittingly, the poor, the elderly, and the disenfranchised have been shut out through no fault of their own, or anyone else's, for that matter. If Canadians want to continue to distinguish their health care system from the American system as a more humane and fair one, they must aggressively target and monitor the have nots of society so that everyone is included in the medicare mix. This disparity has insidiously crept into medicare—now it must be assiduously escorted out.

## QUESTIONS TO ASK

*Although there are a lot of things you cannot control in a hospital, especially during downsizing, there are questions you can ask of the hospital and your family doctor.*

- What is the nursing care like in this hospital?
- What is the nurse-to-bed ratio now? What was it five years ago?
- How long will I have to stay in the hospital?
- What kind of community services are available when I am sent home?
- Will someone come into my home to care for me? If so, do I have to pay for it or is it covered?
- Can I get a list of community services available to me?

## THINGS YOU CAN DO TO HELP

- Demand that governments systematically track the impact of downsizing, especially the impact on the poor and the elderly.
- Advocate that hospitals adequately inform patients of the consequences of downsizing on the services they can–and cannot–provide.

# Conclusion

When I decided to fulfil my lifelong dream of learning how to fly an airplane, I expected the process to be fun and freeing, mixed with some sit-down, textbook work. Early on, my instructor had me practise stalls, spiral dives, spins, landings without engine power, and other emergency procedures. At the time, I was terrified.

I stuck with flying and was licensed as a private pilot in 1996. I realize now that it was important to learn those procedures not just for the impending Transport Canada test, but to do them over and over again until I was no longer frightened and could correct for emergencies quickly, automatically, and without danger to myself or anyone else. Now when I drive to the Toronto Island airport, I feel frightened on the road with other drivers, not in the air with other pilots. At least at the airport, I know the pilots have been tested for their competency. And I know that if I wait more than a month between flights, the flying school that rents me airplanes will have me go back up in the air with an instructor for a "check-out" ride to ensure that I am competent enough to fly their Cessna-172s.

Airline pilots are subjected to even more rigorous standards. At least once a year, with Transport Canada officials looking over their shoulders, they are tested on simulators. "It's not a negotiable thing—they have to meet the standards," said Jock Williams, supervisor of licensing for Transport Canada. "It's a life or death standard. A lack of skills in flying is a smoking hole in the ground"—pilot shorthand for a crashed airliner.

Perhaps the most interesting aspect of aviation regulation is that it not only assumes that errors take place, but it actually prepares fliers for them. That's why all pilots who fly power aircraft, whether for fun or as a career, are taught not only how to correct for mishaps in the air but many other procedures such as fixing high or low approaches on landing, equipment breakdowns, and preventing severe turns from becoming deadly spiral dives. Aware that humans err, pilots are taught how to deal with mistakes.

The aviation philosophy is in direct contrast to that of medicine. Although physicians, nurses, and pharmacists are some of the most careful, conscientious professionals in society, they have a lot of difficulty dealing with mistakes when they do occur. That's largely because the culture of medicine is about being perfect, making the right diagnosis, and not making mistakes, however unrealistic these expectations of infallibility are. In fact, when health care providers do inevitably make an error, there is often a sneaking feeling that they didn't try hard enough.

"Although the notion of infallibility fails the reality test, the fears are well grounded," wrote Harvard School of Public Health professor Dr. Lucian Leape in the *Journal of the American Medical Association*. Oddly, errors in medicine are thought to be the result of a physician's deep character flaw, not a result of being human.

Although physicians discuss their patients' deaths and complications at morbidity and mortality rounds in hospitals, the medical model does not have error prevention built into it. Few accept that wrong doses of medications, incorrect diagnoses, or slips of the scalpel occur often enough that prevention needs to be built into the health care system. Or if they do, little is being done to correct for it. Though every physician intellectually realizes that blunders do occur, the feeling is that one shouldn't criticize a colleague as one's own turn will come next—that somehow it could happen to anyone at any time.

This quest for perfection in medicine creates a strong pressure for those in medicine to cover up mistakes, rather than to admit them. "The organization of medical practice, particularly in the hospital, perpetuates these norms. Errors are rarely admitted or discussed among physicians in private practice … . Far better to conceal a mistake or, if that is impossible, to try to shift the blame to another, even to the patient," Leape wrote.

When an entire medical system makes error-free performance a desirable, even attainable goal, it is doomed to failure, because no system or person is perfect. Even worse, mistakes that occur in that climate are not always quickly noted and rectified. Medical mishaps are such an ugly taboo when they are observed in other arenas of life, some doctors are quick to point fingers. "The media never get it right," some doctors have claimed. When asked for specifics, they inevitably point to the number of corrections published by a given newspaper that day. All reporters, copy editors, and others who put out the paper make mistakes; it's an accepted if undesirable part of the business. Imagine what a safer world it would be if hospitals, doctors, and other health care providers had to publish their errors in a newspaper in front of millions of people.

Perhaps doctors should be compelled to turn in colleagues who have demonstrated improper, incompetent, or substandard behaviour, just as pilots report "near misses" when aircraft have flown too close to them. This requirement for doctors exists in some U.S. states, where a third-party anonymous telephone call from a doctor can prompt an investigation into a fellow physician. In this country, doctors are self-regulating and self-policing, which often means they discipline only the most egregious cases or the baddest apples—not physicians who are only starting to slip. Even when they do, it can take many years for the discipline to come to fruition.

Of all the reasons to admit to mistakes, however, perhaps the strongest one is that telling the truth is the right and ethical thing to do. Johns Hopkins School of Public Health researchers say doctors have an obligation to tell patients about significant medical errors, particularly when such disclosure would benefit the health of the patient, would show respect for the patient's autonomy, or would be called for by principles of justice. "Disclosure should be the rule unless the physician has good reason to sacrifice the patient's autonomy," said lead author Dr. Albert Wu, associate professor of health policy and management at the Baltimore-based university. Perhaps the only exception would be when a severely depressed patient would be incapacitated by the disclosure. In their paper, Wu and other researchers studied individual physician error, rather than system error. They recommended that when a doctor becomes aware of a harmful error made by another doctor, the first physician should encourage the second to disclose the mistake to the patient.

Although disclosing a mistake can lead to the patient becoming angry and upset and even filing a malpractice suit, disclosing an error could also be in the best interests of the doctor, according to Wu. If, for example, the physician admits the error, he or she can take steps to mitigate the damage or take the initiative in recommending a fair, out-of-court settlement. Telling the truth may also strengthen the doctor-patient relationship and perhaps even decrease the likelihood of a lawsuit. "If, on the other hand, a physician does not admit a mistake, the mistake could come to light anyway. Any appearance of a cover-up only increases patient anger and litigiousness," according to a news release issued by Johns Hopkins. Wu suggested that doctors simply state they've made a mistake; "describe in layperson's terms the decisions that were made, including those in which the patient participated; describe the course of events in detail; express personal regret and make a sincere apology. Try not to get defensive and see that financial amends are made."

This book has pointed out many areas where disclosure is not required. Hospitals are not forced to publish their death and complication rates by procedure; nor are they compelled to have minimum volumes of operations to ensure that patients are getting the best and safest care. The cluster of twelve Winnipeg baby deaths may represent an aberration, but who's to say there aren't similar problems with other hospital programs? Since there are no formal, objective monitoring programs in the vast majority of hospitals, patients are worse off because of it—not just because of the care they may receive, but because they can't be informed and do comparison shopping.

Canadians found out about the problems in Winnipeg because the program was shut down and an inquest was subsequently called. Although there are many lessons to learn from Winnipeg, the main ones were those learned by the parents of the dozen dead babies: That a pediatric cardiac program was allowed to form even though some reports had suggested there weren't enough babies to operate on; that a relatively junior surgeon was hired with no senior mentor to help him through the difficulties; that there were complaints from other members of the operating room team that could have been responded to more rapidly. Whatever the inquest findings are in 1999, they will be too late for some families.

If standards similar to those in aviation had been applied

in Winnipeg, the program may not have been able to start because of the low numbers of operations; the surgeon would have to show he was "current" on all procedures and perform a minimum number of them per year to stay that way; and a senior mentor would have been in the "right seat" to watch over the physician and help with difficult areas. The same monitoring could have applied to the rest of the operating room team as well. Finally, when other members of the operating room team complained about what they felt were poor surgical results, there would have been a formal, objective system to deal with their complaints. In the Winnipeg case, whoever was in charge, no one was coming forward to accept responsibility.

If retesting of pilots is important in the aviation industry to make sure they are competent, it should be also required of physicians. Retesting of doctors is routine in the United States, but physicians in Canada are never subject to any tests or competency checks after becoming doctors and specialists. Alberta is expected to be the first province to go ahead with a monitoring program for all of its physicians beginning in fall 1998, said Dr. Larry Ohlhauser, registrar for the College of Physicians and Surgeons of Alberta. The doctor-monitoring program was spearheaded by Ohlhauser, who stated: "I'm a jet pilot and when I go for my ride, I always learn something new." Yet, currently, a doctor can get a licence, not practise for twenty-five years and then put up a shingle the next day.

Some doctors have argued that they can't be compared to pilots. They say the human disease process can't be predicted with the same efficiency as a plane's aerodynamics. But pilots will say that there's nothing more unpredictable than the weather. Both fields are riddled with uncertainty, but rely on a fair amount of science to help them control the things that can be controlled. The real difference is that one industry has error prevention central to its philosophy, making it the safest form of travel. Another difference is that, as Jock Williams, supervisor of licensing for Transport Canada, pointed out: "One high-profile event can really have an impact."

Health care workers rarely have to worry about that kind of high-profile event, largely because their work takes place in the privacy of any one of the 978 hospitals in Canada, not to mention the thousands of doctors' offices, diagnostic centres, and walk-in clinics. Very rarely is there one high-profile event in a hospital that compares to the magnitude of a plane crash.

"The worst airline has to meet minimum standards but the worst hospital doesn't," said Michael Decter, former deputy health minister in Ontario. "In the United States, the thinking is that one-third of physicians are excellent, another third are pretty good, and the last third is pretty bad." Dr. Miles Kilshaw, a consultant from Victoria, points out that "heart surgery mortality rates vary from two per cent to forty per cent. Now if you said eighty of these two hundred people are going die in this plane some of the time, no one would stand for it."

If doctors were subject to routine competency checks as pilots are, it would mean that those who do not make the physician grade would have to go for retraining, or worse, risk losing their jobs. Physicians have the same awesome responsibility pilots do, yet the vast majority of them won't go through as much as one competency check in their entire careers. In aviation, it's called "being current," but the public has no assurances that their physicians are up-to-date in medicine the way pilots are on their aircraft. "I had to meet a standard that validates my competency," said Noble, who flew a DC-8, DC-9, and Boeing-727 during his career.

If one applies the aviation model further, surgeons who learn a new surgical technique would have to perform the operation a required number of "hours" to not only prove their competency but maintain their privileges which, depending on the doctor, allow them to operate and admit patients to hospital. No such high standards were observed in the early 1990s with the rapid adoption of a new technology and operation that promised to revolutionize gall-bladder surgery. Training, in some cases, was poor, with surgeons practising on pigs for a weekend before moving directly to humans under varying amounts of supervision. However, training is much better now and the procedure is considered the best way to remove a gall-bladder.

Transport Canada required David Noble to fly thirty hours on the Airbus-320 every ninety days, but airlines demand even more—they make their pilots log those hours every sixty days. If that was the case for operations, surgeons would have to perform a required number of procedures to maintain their skills. This simple act of ensuring surgeons perform a required number of operations would guarantee they are as "current" as pilots are, thus making it safer for patients going under the knife. The colleges of physicians and surgeons could set volume standards, and hospitals could go one step further, by setting even more stringent ones.

This book has mentioned a number of things hidden from public view about doctors and hospitals, and much has been made of other systems that are superior, particularly in the United States. Certainly, the American health care system, which leaves forty million of its people uninsured, is not better than Canada's. However, the way that Americans collect information, monitor their hospitals and doctors, and publish some good consumer guides is extraordinarily impressive. When this type of information has been published, the death rate drops significantly, surgeons who don't measure up are told to move on, and patients are able to make informed choices.

When Canadians inevitably bring up the impressiveness of these consumer guides, it doesn't take long before someone proposes they are the result of the free-market health care system. The implicit suggestion, of course, is that if Canada wants that type of openness and accountability in its health care system, they will have to buy into the entire U.S. package: a two-tier, private parallel health care system built for the rich. But that is simply not true. Americans have a very strong sense of public safety in their health care system. That, coupled with a strong consumer movement, means they potentially have one of safest health care systems, and the most informed patients in the world. Be they state-mandated laws to publish consumer guides or a toll-free number to check up on doctors, Americans are performing a consumer service unparalleled anywhere else in the world.

That is, with perhaps one exception: the Patient's Charter in Great Britain. The Patient's Charter—something no one else in the world has done—allows for the publishing of hospital report cards using fifty-nine indicators. Patients can see which hospitals meet target times in the emergency ward, how long they will have to queue for a hip replacement, and how long they will have to wait for a specialist's appoint, to name just a few. Publishing the hospital waiting times in Great Britain has meant that long waiting lists have come down. This is attributable to the hospitals trying to get them down, and the government occasionally throwing more money into reducing waiting lists. Even though hospitals still have unusually long waits in some procedures, at least they are tracked—something Canada does not even attempt to do. This is probably one of the greatest public services that could be offered to Canadians: the publishing of waiting lists by surgeon, hospital, and procedure.

The federal government, in coordination with the provincial governments, could create a similar Patient's Charter. By setting standards and targets for waiting times by hospital as Great Britain did, it would not only reduce the inherently long waits for procedures such as hip and knee replacements and cataract surgery, but it would be a big boost to Canadians' confidence in medicare. Patients would finally know there are standards that hospitals are trying to meet, and governments would be compelled to reduce some of the extraordinarily long waits. Patients could also vote with their feet by taking their "business" elsewhere. Waiting lists would cease to be a political club used to beat governments over the head; they would be an accepted part of the system, but not so accepted that inextricably long queues for care would not go unnoticed.

Data could be published as a formal report card sent to Parliament and the provincial legislatures every year. Eventually, they could expand by publishing not only waiting times, but complication and death rates of clinical procedures, such as heart surgery and cancer care, and Caesarean section rates. Ideally, informed patients would be instrumental in helping determine what criteria and procedures should be on the report card on health services.

The Patient's Charter would not only spell out the rights that patients have in the health care system, but would involve follow-up calls to prospective health care consumers, informing them of new changes to legislation or to hospitals. The Charter would have a two-pronged focus: to inform patients of their rights and to educate patients to protect themselves. It wouldn't merely be legislation, but information that health care consumers could use. It would also have the political advantage of helping a public—confused by mixed messages about whether medicare is crumbling—understand that an effort is being made to fix the system.

"What better way to reassure people than to say, 'You

know what? We're going to commit ourselves to a standard of maximum waiting times. We're going to commit ourselves to a level of service against which you can assess us. There are going to be report cards. And we're going to give you meaningful information and it will be up to you to choose,'" said Federal Health Minister Alan Rock in an interview. "I think that would be reassuring to people."

To that end, an audit commission could be established to do routine investigations of hospitals, similar to the one in Great Britain. This audit commission would be funded by the very hospitals it evaluates. Some of the areas this watchdog body could look at during its evaluations include trends such as abnormally high Caesarean section rates and hysterectomy rates, poor rehabilitation following heart attacks, injuries from surgery, or improper prescribing practices. When the investigation is done, the results would be public and hospitals would have no choice but to fix whatever deficiencies had been noted. Both forms of public reporting would keep the focus on waiting times and things that need to be improved in the system, while at the same time providing the added benefit of helping dampen the occasional proposal for two-tier care.

Long waits have been used as a tool to advocate for more money and private care, when one doesn't necessarily have anything to do with the other. In fact, one could argue that if Canadians cannot afford a public system, as some have asserted, then how could they also afford a second, private, parallel health care system? Even though formal, two-tier care does not exist, there are forms of what is called "passive privatization" that seep into the system. The opening for this is usually created by provincial governments that "de-list" medical services under the guise of saving money. However, the only money it saves is in provincial coffers—the cost is of those services is passed directly onto the patient and taxpayers don't get a rebate. Research has shown that when items are de-listed, their prices can rise dramatically. When eye examinations in Alberta were de-listed, the cost of the exams went up by thirty per cent almost immediately.

If Canada's health care system truly is a public system, then provincial governments and doctors' groups should not be able to cut any medical services from provincial health insurance plans without the cuts first being approved by a committee that involves members of the public. In keeping with the theme of accountability, patients or members of the public should not only be heavily involved in any future de-listing, there should also be an annual report of the services cut from provincial health plans.

Certainly, there seems to be a market for private health care in Canada. Some have set up their own private health centres—they can't call them hospitals—in Calgary and Toronto, to name a couple of cities. These businesses are looking at expanding, and while they cannot perform some "medically necessary" procedures such as heart surgery, they do have patients willing to purchase arthroscopy of the knees, rehabilitation, and heart attack prevention programs. No doubt, they are planning for business to get better—something that can only happen as more items are dropped from medicare.

That is not to say that the public, government, and health policy analysts should not be involved in some assessment of what should—and shouldn't be—covered by medicare. It is unrealistic to believe that everything can be covered, mostly because not everything is covered now. Dental bills, prescriptions, and semi-private hospital rooms are just a few areas not insured, with about one-third of all health monies going to the private sector.

Doctors, meanwhile, are being put in the unfair position of having to make difficult choices on who gets care—and who doesn't. These problems exist whenever there are finite resources, particularly when they involve heart operations and knee replacements. One cardiologist I know said he tells his elderly patients they are on the heart surgery list, but not at the "top of the list." That's because as elderly people with other chronic diseases, they are not as good contenders for heart surgery as their middle-aged counterparts. Choices are being made, many by physicians who should not be put in this untenable position. Instead, the public should decide who gets health care and when.

Even when there aren't always clear-cut answers, the Americans have an excellent track record of putting the information out there. This has been seen with the so-called variation rates—a dry term for why more surgeries occur in some counties, regions and countries than others. For decades, equivalent Canadian studies have pointed out that surgeons are removing too many tonsils, adenoids, uteruses, gall-bladders, and other organs, yet nothing is done about it. In the United States, they have tried to solve this problem by publishing the huge differences in rates in consumer guides, which have been very popular. In this country, scientists treat it as a scientific puzzle, arguing that they don't know the "right rate" of surgery so there's not much they can do, other than publish their findings in medical journals where patients can't easily access them.

The philosophy is different in the U.S., as a more consumer-oriented society. The thinking of their scientists is that the only "right rate" of surgery is the one informed health care consumers make by having information on areas where they are most likely to get their organs removed. With few exceptions, there has been no widescale attempt to inform the public of the huge differences in surgical rates in Canada.

Notwithstanding those problems, there are some who are trying in their own way to enhance the quality in their hospitals by setting up programs, encouraging doctors to follow treatment guidelines, and clamping down on those who fall below medical benchmarks. One can't help but look at the impressive cancer survival rates in British Columbia and be impressed. That province has some of the highest survival rates of various types of cancer, including that of the breast, which they attribute to having a policy manual that is distributed to all doctors who treat the many diseases that make up cancer. This is a Canadian success story, and despite all those who question whether guidelines are really effective, B.C. has a greater survival rate to back up their claims.

At Toronto Hospital, there is an internal quality program

that scrutinizes death rates, readmission rates, and infection rates by department and by individual doctor. "We look at when benchmarks are broken and why," said Dr. Paul Walker, surgeon-in-chief at Toronto Hospital. "You can get overwhelmed with these oversick [very ill] patients nobody wants to do." For example, one of the many things the hospital tracks are infections following surgery. The Orthopedic Business Unit of the hospital reported in April 1995 that it had 36 infections out of 1610 cases for a 2.24 per cent infection rate. Since the threshold is one to five per cent, that's considered excellent. "If I can't defend what I'm doing or talk about it, then I'm not in good shape," Walker said of his figures. "As a doctor, you have to be able to be questioned. It's not fair if people are given too little information. I'm a great believer in having patients know what's going on. We have a great deal of information we give patients."

Toronto Hospital's Dr. Tirone David, chief of cardiovascular surgery, routinely examines the death rates and infection rates of the cardiac surgeons in his department through a data program that costs $150,000 a year to operate. In one case, a doctor had a 18.8 per cent death rate that couldn't be explained by a complicated case-mix of severely ill heart patients alone. In his eight years as chief of cardiovascular surgery, David has encouraged three training heart surgeons to move on. While the doctors were not poor at their jobs, they weren't up to the hospital's high standards, either. "We set a higher standard here," said David, reputed to be one of the world's great heart surgeons.

He said there is "enormous variation" among the abilities of surgeons. "In [the city of] Toronto, there are reasonable surgeons. Are they shining stars? Few are."

The Canadian Council on Health Services Accreditation, which accredits hospitals, is also starting to get into the measurement act. Long criticized for being too soft on hospitals, the organization is beginning to look at the idea of having clinical scorecards for hospitals. "We're setting ourselves a target of the year 2000. We're looking for a set of indicators that could be recommended to all health care organizations," said Elma Heidemann, executive director of the council. The council is planning to create a hospital record that could include its performance on cancer care, Caesarean section rates, and the time patients wait in the emergency room before being admitted to a bed. "Everybody's keen—everybody sees the value of doing this," Heidemann said.

At the University of Toronto, professors George Pink, Sandy Leggat, and Michael Murray are doing a balanced scorecard on eleven Toronto hospitals with an eye to finding variations in management practices, in addition to tracking patient satisfaction and finance. "In the United States, there's a data-driven approach. That's where we really fall down in Canada," said Pink. In Canada, doctors often complain the data are not good enough so they shouldn't be measured, but Murray points out that "we're never going to have perfect enough data." Ted Freedman, chief executive officer of Toronto's Mount Sinai Hospital, who is also involved in the project, said "hospitals have been strange institutions in that we couldn't tell you accurately the cost of the product. You didn't have to—someone gave you a pot of money." Only now "has there been a general acceptance that funding should be related to efficiency," he said.

Certainly, it appears that some are getting into the measurement act, with the creation of hospital report cards. In 1997, the Oakville-Trafalgar Memorial Hospital board of governors passed a resolution that was later adopted at the Ontario Hospital Association's (OHA) annual meeting. It said the OHA will "undertake to develop appropriate comparative indicators which will allow residents in Ontario's communities to make informed choices with respect to the outcomes and level of quality being provided by hospitals in Ontario." The resolution, the last of six passed by the OHA, said it "is important for residents of their communities to be able to make informed choices when seeking care from hospitals" and that "meaningful and objective indicators of outcomes and quality of services would be of assistance to people who are making decisions about choice of hospital and physician."

According to David MacKinnon, president of the OHA, these indicators are to be translated into annual report cards for the province's hospitals in what could be a first in Canada. "We think this is very important in terms of giving the public confidence," Geoff McKenzie, chair of Toronto's Riverdale Hospital and chair of OHA, told *Toronto Star* reporter Art Chamberlain. "There is nothing more important to the consumer than the quality of health care.

Other industries all provide information, in one way or another, on their performance, but in health care we don't." Although the *Toronto Star* welcomed the announcement in an editorial, it had a note of caution: "The OHA must assure the public that it can produce a credible, useful annual report. Otherwise, we may need the equivalent of Britain's independent Audit Commission, which tracks problems in the health care system and publishes the results."

Improvements in the health care system aren't exclusive to Ontario. In Saskatchewan, the Health Services Utilization and Research Commission goes a step further than many scientific bodies that study health care practices: It actually gets doctors to change their behaviour. Not satisfied merely to pump out research in journals, this group also surveys doctors to finds out what would help physicians in their practices. In that province, electrocardiograms (ECGs) declined thirteen per cent over three years after guidelines on when to use them were distributed to doctors. "The ECGs alone saved $600,000 a year for guides that cost us $50,000 a year to produce," said its chief executive officer Steven Lewis. And that's just one of many examples. As Lewis points out, "it's foolish to collect data if there is no strategy to put it into place."

A number of themes emerge in Canada's health care system: There is no accountability to patients and taxpayers; there is little information publicly available so that patients can make informed decisions; and the job has been left to doctors and hospitals under the motto "we know best." Patients believed the self-regulated system was working, while many others assumed that because government wrote the cheques that was somehow the equivalent of a seal of medical approval. Many others were intimidated by the elitist language of the medical world, which wasn't keen to have them take part in treatment decisions. They grudgingly accepted the paternalism of the medical system.

In their eagerness to provide care to all, Canadians haven't thought much about how good, bad, or necessary that care is: As long as it was being provided, that was good enough. As long as equal access was provided, there was an assumption, even an expectation, that no one was left out and that care was excellent. Despite the best of intentions, this standard has not been met. If the system is to change, which indeed it must, then patients' expectations may also have to change.

Building accountability into the health care system is about accepting, even expecting, that surgical slips, medication errors, or even a lack of nursing care are going to occur. Accountability is about being real, fallible, and understanding that doctors and hospitals do not have all the answers. It's about letting patients take a big part in their health care decisions—not designing their treatment, but certainly being fully informed about it. If Canadians are ready for accountability, there is going to be a trade-off in the form of a different kind of doctor working in the world of medicine, an uncertain mix of science and art. Answers aren't always clear-cut. That will be an adjustment for everyone, but it will probably sit well with many patients, particularly if there is something to be gained from it.

Although piecemeal approaches are being made, it is going to take a strong consumer movement—individually and collectively—to make the health care system strong, accountable, and safe. Canadians should do to their health care system what Ralph Nader did to the American automobile industry by ensuring that proper controls and standards are in place to make it the safest, best industry there is.

Collectively, this can be done by lobbying provincial and federal governments for report cards, publishing death and complication rates, making it easier for hospitals to shed low-volume programs and substandard physicians, and the creation of a Patient's Charter similar to Great Britain's. Politicians—both federally and provincially—would act if patients and taxpayers made enough demands to revamp medicare and if a consumer movement was born. Politicians would have no choice but to fix the social program Canadians cherish the most.

Every day there isn't accountability in the health care system, a pregnant woman doesn't know which hospital she is most likely to get a Caesarean section in; a parent isn't sure where to take their ailing child for a given operation; and a heart patient can't find out which cardiac surgeon he or she is most likely to survive under. Women have their uteruses removed when they should have drug therapy, and elderly women are admitted to hospital for drug reactions because they've been written one too many prescriptions for mood-altering pills. More patients die from cancer than need to. And some patients who get operations are injured and can't get compensation. Others languish unnecessarily on waiting lists, unaware which hospital or surgeon has the shortest queuing times for care. Some never make even make it that far, as they fall off the edge of care and don't get operations or treatment and are none the wiser. Many others have excellent care and are pleased with the result.

Information, planning for error, and informing patients are the keys to fixing medicare. And the best way to do that is with the publishing of consumer guides, report cards, and an objective system that roots out those providing substandard care. These are not heady aspirations—they are the basics that should be provided to prospective patients and taxpayers.

Health care consumers need to know that someone is in charge; that someone will regulate hospitals and doctors in a way that is not only safe, but that provides the best possible care. For patients, it means they are still in the passenger's seat, but that doesn't mean they can't shop around for the best airline with the top safety record. Being informed and having tough standards and a good aviation record has helped take the fear out of flying for many.

More of us use hospitals and doctors than fly in airplanes. If there is one thing all Canadians share universally over and over again, it is their use of the health care system. But we don't demand anywhere near the same safety standards for doctors, hospitals, and health centres that we do for pilots and airlines. Others have mistakenly assumed that those standards are already in hospitals because the government funds the health care system. But the government is an insurer, not a watchdog—it merely writes the cheques. If similar standards were applied to the health care system and prospective patients could shop around, there would be little for patients to fear at the hospital or doctor's office. After all, getting sick is frightening, but getting medical treatment shouldn't be.

# Selected Bibliography

Hundreds of books, articles, and studies were consulted during the course of writing this book. Although many of them were cited in the text, you may be interested in further reading on the subject of health care accountablilty, quality, and consumer report cards.

Anderson, G.M. *Hospital Restructuring and Epidemiology of Hospital Utilization.* Medical Care 35, 10, Supplement.

Anderson, G.M., Grumbach, K., Luft, H.S., et al. *Use of coronory artery bypass surgery in the United States and Canada. Influence of age and outcome.* Journal of the American Medical Association 269 (1993): 1661-66.

*Cancer Surgery Practice Atlas: Cancer Surgery in Ontario.* Toronto: Institute for Clinical Evaluative Sciences in Ontario, 1997: 254.

Chassin, M.R., Hannan, E.L., DeBuono, B.A. *Benefits and*

*hazards of reporting medical outcomes publicly.* New England Journal of Medicine 334 (1996): 394-98.

Cohen, M.M., Young, W., Theriault, M.E., Hernandez, R. *Has laparoscopic cholecystectomy changed patterns of practice and patient outcome in Ontario?* Canadian Medical Association Journal 154, 4 (1996): 491-500.

Decter, M. *Managing Health System Change the Canadian Way.* Toronto: McGilligan Books, 1994: 260.

Delamothe, T. *Outcomes into Clinical Practice.* London, England: BMJ Publishing Group, 1994: 169.

Deziel, D.J., Millikan, K.W., Economou, S.G., Doolas, K., Ko, S.T., Airan, M.C. *Complications of laparoscopic cholecystectomy: a national survey of 4,292 hospitals and analysis of 77,604 cases.* The American Journal of Surgery 165, 1 (1993): 9-14.

Dyck, F., et al. *Effect of Surveillance on the number of hysterectomies in the province of Saskatchewan.* New England Journal of Medicine 296 (1977): 1326.

Dziuban, S., McIlduff, J., Miller, J., Dal Col, R. *How a New York Cardiac Surgery Program Uses Outcomes Data. Albany, N.Y.* Annals of Thoracic Surgery 58 (1994): 1871-76.

Epstein, A. *Performance reports on quality: prototypes, problems, and prospects.* New England Journal of Medicine 333 (1995): 57-61.

Escarce, J.J., Shea, J.A., Schwartz, J.S. *How Practicing Surgeons Trained for Laparoscopic Cholecystectomy.* Medical Care 35, 3: 291-96.

Ghali, W., Ash, A., Hall, R., Mokowitz, M. *Statewide Quality Improvement Initiatives and Mortality After Cardiac Surgery.* Journal of the American Medical Association 277 (1997): 379-82.

Green, J., Wintfeld, N. *Report cards on cardiac surgeons: Assessing New York State's approach.* New England Journal of Medicine 332 (1995): 1229-32.

Green, J., Wintfeld, N., Krasner, M., Wells, C. *In search of America's best hospitals: The promise and reality of quality assessment.* Journal of the American Medical Association 277 (1997): 1152-55.

Hannan, E.L., Bernard, H.R., Kilburn, H.C., O'Donnell, J.F. *Gender differences in mortality rates of coronary artery bypass surgery.* American Heart Journal 123 (1992): 866-72.

Hannan, E.L., Kumar, D., Racz, M., Siu, A.L., Chassin, M.R. *New York State's Cardiac Surgery Reporting System: Four years later.* Annals of Thoracic Surgery 58 (1994): 1852-57.

Hannan, E.L., Kilburn, H. Jr., Racz, M., Shields, E., Chassin, M.R. *Improving the outcomes of coronary artery bypass surgery in New York State.* Journal of the American Medical Association 271 (1994): 761-66.

Hannan, E., Siu, A., Kumar, D., et al. *The Decline in Coronary Artery Bypass Graft Surgery Mortality in New York State: The Role of Surgeon Volume.* Journal of the American Medical Association 273 (1995): 209-13.

Hayward, R., Guyatt, G., Moore, K., et al. *Canadian physicians' attitudes about preference regarding clinical practice guidelines.* Canadian Medical Association of Journal 156, 12 (June 15, 1997).

Higginson, L., Cairns, J., Smith, E. *Rates of cardiac catheterization, coronary angioplasty and coronary artery bypass surgery in Canada [1991].* Canadian Journal of Cardiology 10, 7 (September 1994).

Hope, T. *Evidence-Based Patient Choice.* London, England: King's Fund Publishing, 1996: 39.

Joffres, M.R., et al. *Awareness, treatment and control of hypertension in Canada.* American Journal of Hypertension 10 (1997): 1097-1102.

Land, G., Longo, D.R., Hoskins, B., Fraas, J. *The development of a consumer guide on the quality of obstetrical services: The Missouri experience.* Journal of Public Health Management Practice 1 (1995): 35-43.

Leape, L. *Error in Medicine.* Journal of the American Medical Association 272, 23 (December 21, 1994).

Leatt, P., Pink, G., Naylor, D. *Integrated Delivery Systems: Has their time come in Canada?* Canadian Medical Association Journal 154, 6 (1996).

Leslie, K.A., Rankin, R.N., Duff, J.H. *Lost gallstones during laparoscopic cholecystectomy: Are they really benign?* Canadian Journal of Surgery 37 (1994): 240-42.

Macho, J., Cable, G. *Everyone's Guide to Outpatient Surgery.* Toronto: Somerville House Publishing, 1996:185.

Mickleborough, L., Tagaki, Y., Maruyama, H. *Is Sex a Factor in Determining Operative Risk for Aortocoronary Bypass Graft Surgery? Supplement II.* Circulation 92, 9 (November 1, 1995).

Naylor, D., Williams, J.I., et al. *Primary hip and knee replacement surgery: Ontario criteria for case selection and surgical priority.* Quality in Health Care 5 (1996): 20-30.

Nenner, R.P., Imperato, P.J., Will, T.O., et al. *Hospital reported complications of laparoscopic cholecystectomy among Medicare and Medicaid patients.* Journal of Community Health 18 (1993): 253-60.

New York State Department of Health. *Coronary Artery Bypass Surgery.* Albany, NY: New York State Department of Health, 1996: 17.

Nightingale, F. *Notes on Nursing: What It Is and What It Is Not.* New York, NY: Dover Publications, 1969.

O'Malley, Martin. *Hospital: Life and Death in a Major Medical Centre.* Toronto: Macmillan of Canada, 1986.

Park, R.E., Brook, R.H., Kosecoff, J., et al. *Explaining variations in hospital death rates: Randomness, severity of illness, quality of care.* Journal of the American Medical Association 264 (1990): 484-90.

*Patterns of Health Care in Ontario, 1st ed.* Toronto: Institute for Clinical Evaluative Sciences in Ontario, 1994: 329.

*Patterns of Health Care in Ontario, 2nd ed.* Toronto: Institute for Clinical Evaluative Sciences in Ontario, 1996: 354.

Patterson, E., Nagy, G. *Don't cry over spilled stones? Complications of gallstones spilled during laparoscopic cholecystectomy: Case report and literature review.* Canadian Journal of Surgery 40, 4 (1997): 300-304.

The Pennsylvania Health Care Cost Containment Council. *A Consumer Guide to Coronary Artery Bypass Graft Surgery.* Harrisburg: The Pennsylvania Health Care Cost Containment Council, 1995: 48.

*Questions and Answers on Breast Cancer: A guide for women and their physicians.* Ottawa: Canadian Medical Association, 1998: 31.

Rachlis, M., Kushner, C. *Second Opinion: What's Wrong with Canada's Health Care System.* Toronto: HarperCollins, 1989: 371.

Rachlis, M., Kushner, C. *Strong Medicine: How to Save Canada's Health Care System.* Toronto: HarperCollins, 1994: 396.

Rouleau, J.L., Moye, L.A., Pfeffer, M.A., et al. *A comparison of management patterns after acute myocardial infarction in Canada and the United States.* New England Journal of Medicine 328 (1993): 779-84.

Schneider, E., Epstein, A. *Influence of Cardiac-Surgery Performance Reports on Referral Practices and Access to Care: A Survey of Cardiovascular Specialists.* New England Journal of Medicine 335 (1996): 251-56.

Shea, J.A., Healey, M.J., Berlin, J.A., et al. *Mortality and Complications Associated with Laparoscopic Cholecystectomy: A Meta-Analysis.* Annals of Surgery 224, 5: 609-620.

*Show Me Buyer's Guide: Outpatient Procedures.* Jefferson City: Missouri Department of Health, 1994 and 1995.

*Show Me Buyer's Guide: Obstetrical Services.* Jefferson City: Missouri Department of Health, 1994.

Simmons, H.E. *The Nation's Least Understood Health Care Problem—The Quality of Medical Care.* Generations (Summer 1996).

Smith, G. White, Naifeh, S. *Making Miracles Happen.* Boston: Little, Brown and Company, 1997: 320.

The Southern Surgeons Club. *A prospective analysis of 1518 laparoscopic cholecystectomies.* New England Journal of Medicine 324 (1991): 1073-78.

Starr, Paul. *The Social Trasnformation of American Medicine.* New York: Basic Books, 1982.

*Survey of Routine Maternity Care and Practices in Canadian*

*Hospitals, 1st ed.* Ottawa: Canadian Institute of Child Health, 1995: 236.

Tarbox, B.B., Rockwood, J.K., Abernathy, C.M. *Are modified radical mastectomies done for T1 breast cancer because of surgeon's advice or patient's choice?* American Journal of Surgery 164 (1992): 417-20.

Targarona, E.M., Balagué, C., Cifuentes, A., Martinez, J., Trias, M. *The spilled stone: A potential danger after laparoscopic cholecystectomy [review].* Surgical Endoscopy 9, 7 (1995): 768-73.

Taylor, B. *Common bile duct injury during laparoscopic cholecystectomy in Ontario: Does ICD-9 coding indicate true incidence?* Canadian Medical Association Journal 158, 4 (1998).

U.S. Congress, Office of Technology Assessment. *The Quality of Medical Care: Information for Consumers.* Washington, DC: Office of Technology Assessment, 1988.

U.S. News & World Report. *America's Best Hospitals.* New York: John Wiley & Sons Inc., 1996: 508.

Vayda, E. *A comparison of surgical rates in Canada and in England and Wales.* New England Journal of Medicine 289 (1973): 1224-29.

Weiler, P.C., Hiatt, H.H., Newhouse, H.P., et al. *A Measure of Malpractice: Medical Injury, Malpractice Litigation, and Patient Compensation.* Cambridge, Massachusetts: Harvard University Press, 1993: 177.

Wetscher, G., Schwab, G., Fend, F., Glaser, K., Ladurner, D., Bodner, E. *Subcutaneous abscess due to gallstones lost during laparoscopic cholecystectomy.* Endoscopy 26, 3 (1994): 324-25.

Wright, J., Sunshine, L. *The Best Hospitals in America: The Top Rated Medical Facilities in the U.S. and Canada.* Detroit: Visible Ink Press, 1995: 609.

York, Geoffrey. *The High Price of Health: A Patient's Guide to the Hazards of Medical Politics.* Toronto: Lorimer, 1987.

# Index

## M



## N



## O

## S



## T